Album of Malaria

from Hyperendemicity to Elimination in Yunnan

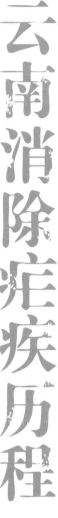

云南消除疟疾历程

— 主编 —

周红宁　许建卫　林祖锐

云南出版集团

YNK 云南科技出版社

·昆明·

图书在版编目（CIP）数据

云南消除疟疾历程 / 周红宁, 许建卫, 林祖锐主编
. -- 昆明：云南科技出版社, 2021.12
ISBN 978-7-5587-4057-2

Ⅰ.①云… Ⅱ.①周… ②许… ③林… Ⅲ.①疟疾—防治—云南 Ⅳ.①R531.3

中国版本图书馆CIP数据核字(2021)第259951号

云南消除疟疾历程
YUNNAN XIAOCHU NÜEJI LICHENG

周红宁　许建卫　林祖锐　主编

出 版 人：温　翔
策　　划：高　亢　刘　康
责任编辑：马　莹　叶佳林
整体设计：长策文化
责任校对：张舒园
责任印制：蒋丽芬

书　　号：ISBN 978-7-5587-4057-2
印　　刷：昆明亮彩印务有限公司
开　　本：889mm×1194mm　1/16
印　　张：6
字　　数：180千字
版　　次：2021年12月第1版
印　　次：2021年12月第1次印刷
定　　价：168.00元

出版发行：云南出版集团　云南科技出版社
地　　址：昆明市环城西路609号
电　　话：0871-64192372

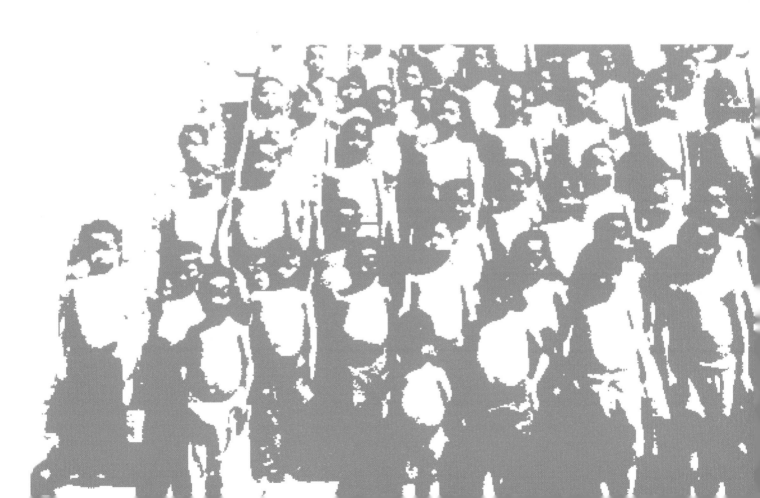

序

疟疾主要是一种经按蚊传播，由疟原虫引起的古老寄生虫病。疟原虫主要寄生于人类血液红细胞和肝细胞等细胞中，疟原虫在血液内大量繁殖，破坏红细胞而引起寒战、发热，并伴有头痛、乏力等典型的临床症状，救治不及时常引起重症或致人死亡。目前全球100多个国家存在疟疾流行，每年约2亿人感染疟疾，50万人死亡，其中90%疟疾病例主要发生在非洲，特别是撒哈拉以南地区。

疟疾从一开始就与人类文明如影随形。在我国，早在殷墟甲骨文中就已有"疟"字的记载。传染病在我国古代医籍中记载最详者首推疟疾。英文中的"疟疾"一词源于意大利语，意为"坏空气"。云南解放前也把疟疾称"瘴气"，民间普遍把疟疾发作叫"打摆子"。

云南省地处我国西南边陲，属"少、边、山、穷"社会经济欠发达地区，西南部与疟疾严重的缅甸、老挝和越南毗连，国境长4 060千米。地形地貌和自然环境复杂，多种气候类型并存，导致传疟媒介种类众多且复杂，容易引起疟疾传播或流行。这些自然地理和社会经济特点使得云南成为我国疟疾流行最严重、控制和消除最困难的省份。如1953年，全省共报告疟疾病例41万多例，发病率248.36/万，占20世纪90年代前全省传染病总数的60%。

解放后，云南疟疾防治工作在党和政府的关怀、领导下，历经70余年，通过几代疟防工作者的努力拼搏，2008年全省疟疾发病率控制到万分之一以下，2015年5月实现无本地感染的恶性疟疾病例，2016年5月至今持续保持无本土感染的疟疾病例状态。2020年1月通过国家消除疟疾技术评估，2020年6月通过国家消除疟疾终审评估。2021年6月30日，我国获得了WHO无疟疾国家的认证。这也结束了疟疾严重危害全省人民健康的历史，为全省人民健康事业和社会经济发展做出卓越贡献。

本着尊重和再现云南省解放前、解放后消除疟疾历史的原则，本书收集了各个时期珍贵的历史图片，并按时间顺序编排。全书采用图文并茂的形式，分解放前疟疾流行和防治（1950年以前，"云南解放日"为 1950年2月24日）、疟疾流行基线调查与防治试点、控制疟疾发病率、疟疾大幅回升与控制暴发流行、降低发病率和巩固扩大防治成果和消除疟疾六个部分，充分展示了云南几代疟疾防治工作者的无私奉献和顽强抗疟的风采，以及云南疟疾从高度地方性流行到消除的历史画面。相信本书的出版，能继续激励现今或将来疟疾防治工作者以前辈为榜样，努力拼搏，以更严谨的科学态度、更扎实过硬的技术，防止输入疟疾再传播，为健康云南和云南周边国家2030年消除疟疾再立新功。

Preface

Malaria is an ancient *Plasmodium* sp. disease that is mainly transmitted by Anopheline mosquitoes. *Plasmodium* mainly infests human red blood cells and liver cells. The malaria parasites undergo a massive cellular division in red blood cells，then destroy the red cells to cause clinical symptoms such as chills, fever, headache, and general weakness. Untimely treatment often leads to severe or fatal illness. At present, malaria remains endemic in more than 100 countries in the world. Approximately 200 million people are infected with malaria, and about 500 thousand people die of it per year. 90% of these malaria incidence and death occur in Africa, particularly in the Sub-Saharan.

Malaria has been closely accompanying human civilization from the very beginning. In China, the word "nüè" (malaria) was recorded in the oracle bone inscriptions Yin Xu. The most well-recorded infectious disease in ancient Chinese medical texts is malaria. The English word "malaria" is derived from the Italian for "bad air". In Yunnan, malaria was also called "bad air" before 1950 and malaria symptoms were commonly referred to as "Da Bai Zi" in folklore.

Yunnan Province is located in the southwest border of China, and its 4 060-kilometer southwestern border is contiguous with malaria-endemic countries such as Myanmar, Laos and Vietnam. Yunnan is a province of "ethnic minority, border, being mountainous and poverty-stricken". Under the complex topographical and environmental conditions along with multiple coexisting climate types, the malaria-transmitting vectors thrive in variety and complexity of species, making it easy for malaria to transmit or become prevalent. The underdeveloped situation in the socioeconomic aspect, and naturally geographical and socio-economic factors decided that Yunnan was an area with malaria hyperendemicity. It was the most difficult province to control and eliminate malaria in China. In 1953, the number of reported malaria cases was over 410 thousand, and the malaria incidence was as high as 24.838 per 1 000 person-years. Malaria accounted for 60% of the total number of infectious diseases in the Province prior to 1990s.

After liberation, under the solicitude and leadership of the Communist Party and the governments at each level, as a results of healthcare workers' intergenerational hard work and intensive efforts for more than 70 years, malaria prevention and control have obtained a great achievement. In the whole province, malaria incidence rate was controlled under 0.1 per 1 000 person-years in 2008; achieved and maintained *Plasmodium falciparum* malaria free since May 2015, and then zero indigenous cases for malaria since May 2016. Yunnan Province had passed the national technical assessment in January 2020, and then the final national malaria elimination assessment in June. At last, the World Health Organization certificated China as malaria-free on 30 June 2021.The achieved goal of malaria-free terminated the history of malaria rampancy in Yunnan, which was seriously endangering people's health. The achievement also contributed outstandingly to people's health and socioeconomic development in the Province.

In accordance with the principle of respecting and reproducing the history of eliminating malaria in Yunnan Province before and after liberation, this book collects and chronologically displays precious historical photos from various periods. It is in an illustrated format and contains six parts, namely, malaria prevalence and control before liberation (prior to 24 February 1950, the Day of Yunnan Liberation), baseline survey and pilot control trials, controlling the incidence of malaria, malaria resurgence and outbreak control, consolidating and scaling up achievement and eliminating malaria. This book presents the full historical profile of malaria from hyperendemicity to elimination in Yunnan, and fully reveals the selfless dedication and tenacious acts of healthcare workers for generations. It is believed that the publication of this book will certainly encourage people who are working in the field of malaria control at every level now and future by following the examples of their predecessors to work hard with rigorous scientific attitude, solid and excellent techniques to fight the disease, to prevent reintroduction of malaria in Yunnan to contribute to "Healthy Yunnan" and also malaria elimination in neighboring countries by 2030.

Contents
目录

1944
1945
1946
1947
1948
1949
1950
1951
1952
1953
1954
1955
1956
1957
1958
1959
1960
1961
1962
1963
1964
1965
1966
1967
1968
1969
1970
1971
1972
1973
1974
1975
1976
1977
1978
1979
1980
1981
1982
1983
1984
1985
1986
1987
1988
1989
1990
1991
1992
1993
1994
1995
1996
1997
1998
1999
2000
2001
2002
2003
2004
2005
2006
2007
2008
2009
2010
2011
2012
2013
2014
2015
2016
2017
2018
2019
2020

1950

1955

1970

1985

2010

2020

Part 1
Malaria Epidemics and Control
Before Liberation

民间老话 "要到思茅坝/潞西坝/盈江坝，先把老婆嫁"，是解放前云南疟疾流行严重的真实写照。意思是"到海拔较低的地区容易感染疟疾及死亡，去之前最好先把老婆嫁了，以免她守寡"。因解放前，云南缺乏防疫机构，没有疟疾发病和流行程度的统计数据。仅是相传1904—1910年滇越铁路从修建到通车期间，10万死亡民工中多数死于疟疾（有的文章报告死亡20万人，《云南铁路始末》记载为死亡6万~7万人，法国印度支那铁路建设公司的 *The manual of Yunnan Railway Line* 则记载仅死亡12 000人）。其次，1919—1949年思茅疟疾流行，思茅坝区常住人口从1919年的7万余人锐减到1949年的2 000人以下。1933—1940年，云县疟疾大流行，导致33 000人死亡。

清代及之前，由于云南缺乏基本的卫生服务系统，治疗疟疾主要采用民间中医或草药，以及诉诸鬼神等方法。民国时期，虽有政府医疗服务机构，亦取得一定效果，但收效甚微，无法抵挡疟疾在云南的肆虐。如1935年1月思茅人后晋修（上海东南医科大学毕业生、云南陆军医院医生），应家乡40余人联名请求回乡成立了思普医院并开展抗疟活动；当时他亲手制作蚊子模型彩灯向民众宣传抗疟知识，通过调查发现，思茅当时疟疾发病率高达72.88%；但由于当地付不起医院职工工资，最终后晋修于当年11月返回昆明，民国时期思茅最后一次抗疟失败。为确保抗日战争的后勤保障，修建滇

图 1.1~1.4

1904—1910年滇越铁路工地现场，民工工作和生活情况，建成的"人"字桥。铁路修建过程中约10万民工死于疟疾、饥饿和工头暴力，可谓"一根枕木一条命，一颗道钉一滴血"。

Fig. 1.1-1.4

Yunnan-Vietnam Railway construction site 1904-1910: the working and living conditions of workers; the completed bridge that looked like the Chinese character for "human". About 100 thousand of workers died of malaria, hunger and foreman's abuse during the construction of the railway. It can be said, "a railway crosstie, a human life; a railway spike, a drop of human blood".

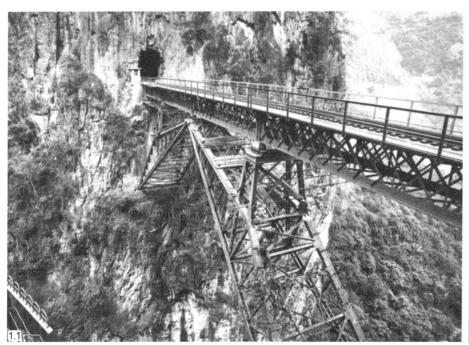

1.1

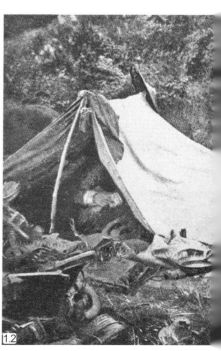

1.2

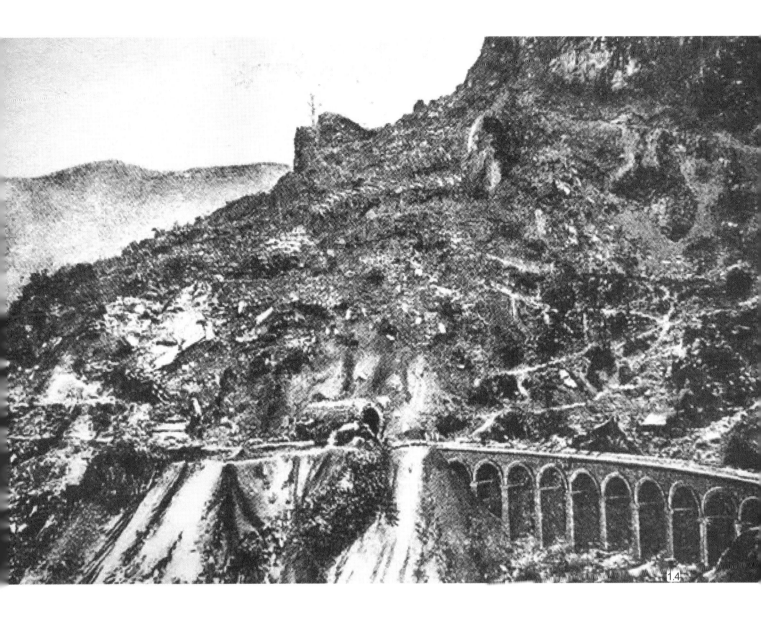

1.4

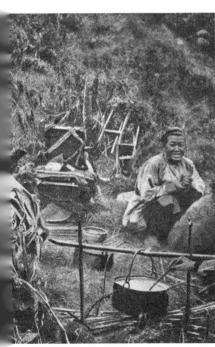

1.3

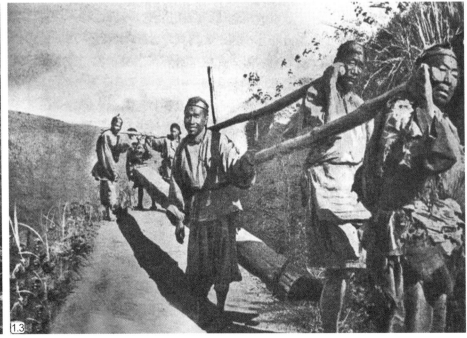

第一部分
解放前疟疾流行和防治

缅铁路（1938—1942年），1939年云南全省抗疟委员会开始在云县等地开展抗疟工作，向公路建筑员工和当地群众定期发放奎宁片和阿的平等抗疟药品，使云县等地死亡人数逐步减少，但疟疾仍然较流行，如1940年疟疾专家郑祖佑医生在云县的疟疾调查结果显示，当地疟疾引起脾肿率还高达94.1%（4 766/5 069），疟原虫带虫率高达50.7%（2 566/5 069）。

The folk saying "Marry out your wife first if you want to go to the lowland of Simao, Luxi or Yingjiang" was a true reflection of the grave malaria epidemic in Yunnan before liberation, which means that if you go to a lower altitude area where you are prone to malaria and death, you'd better marry out your wife before you leave home, so that your wife would not be widowed. However, there was no statistical data of malaria incidence and prevalence due to lack of a complete health service system. It was only rumored: from 1904 to 1910, about 100 thousand of deaths occurred during the construction of the Yunnan-Vietnam Railway, and most of them died of malaria (200 thousand deaths in some records, 60-70 thousand deaths in the book *Beginning and Ending of Yunnan–Vietnam Railway*, but only 12 000 deaths in *The Manual of Yunnan Railway Line* edited by the French Indo-China Railway Construction Co.). Additionally, during the 1919-1949 malaria epidemic in Simao, the resident population of Simao dam area plummeted from more than 70 000 in 1919 to less than 2 000 in 1949. Third, the epidemic of malaria in Yunxian County from 1933 to 1940 resulted in 33 000 deaths.

图 1.5~1.6

思茅疟疾流行后1950年3月杂草丛生的街道和1910年前后繁华的街景。据说，"疟疾流行初期，每户可免死，但不免病；继而每户可免死绝，但不免有死亡；后来疫情越来越严重，有的全家、全寨和整条街死绝"。

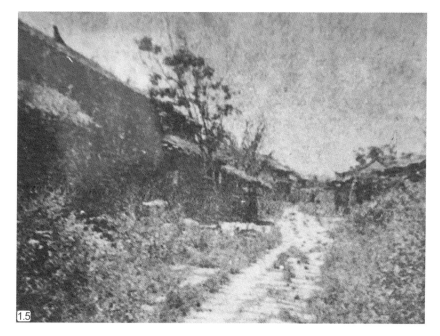

1.5

Fig. 1.5-1.6

The weedy and bushy street of Simao after the malaria epidemic in March 1950, in contrast to the busy street around 1910. It is said that "In the early stage of the epidemic, every household could be free from death; but not from the disease; later, a household could avoid annihilation, but not death; and then the epidemic became more and more serious at last, in some cases the all family members, the whole village and the whole street died out".

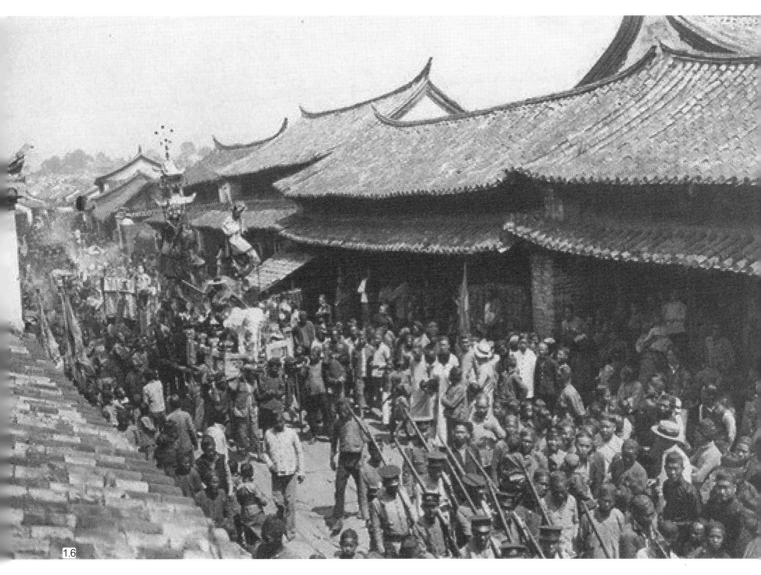

1.6

Public health service system was basically unavailable in Yunnan during the Qing Dynasty and before. Malaria was treated mainly by traditional Chinese medicine or herbal medicine, or by appealing to ghosts and gods. During the period of the Republic of China, although there were public health service institutions that were available and somewhat effective, but the interventions could not effectively control rampant malaria, so the impact was rather limited. In January 1935, a native of Simao, Hou Jinxiu (a graduate of Shanghai Southeast Medical University and a doctor at Yunnan Army Hospital), at the request of more than 40 people from his hometown, returned to his birthplace to set up the Sipu Hospital and carry out anti-malaria activities; at that time, he personally made mosquito figure lanterns to promote anti-malaria knowledge to the public. Through investigation, he found that the incidence of malaria in Simao was as high as 72.88%. However, because of the lack of funding to pay for the staff of the Hospital, Dr. Hou had to return to Kunming in November of the same year, so the Kuomintang Government lost the final fight against malaria in Simao. In order to ensure logistical support for the Anti-Japanese War, the Yunnan-Burma Railway (1938-1942) was built, and Yunnan Provincial Committee of Malaria Control began to implement antimalarial interventions in Yunxian County and other places along the railway construction sites in 1939. Antimalarial drugs such as quinine and quinacrine tablets were regularly distributed to the railway construction workers and also local residents. The intervention gradually reduced the malaria deaths. However, malaria incidence and prevalence was still high, for example, the results of investigation conducted by malaria expert Dr. Zheng Zuyou in Yunxian County in 1940, showed that the spleen rate caused by malaria was still as high as 94.1% (4 766/5 069) and the Plasmodium parasite rate as high as 50.7% (2 566/5 069) .

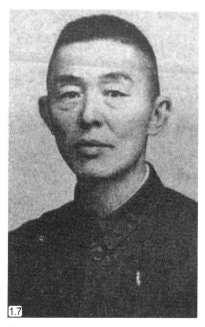

图 1.7

后晋修医生，1935年1—11月在思茅成立思普医院开展疟疾控制活动，但因缺乏经费和物资功败垂成。

Fig. 1.7

Dr. Hou, who established the Simao-Pu'er Hospital to carry out malaria control activities from January to November 1935, but lost his project due to shortage of funding and supplies.

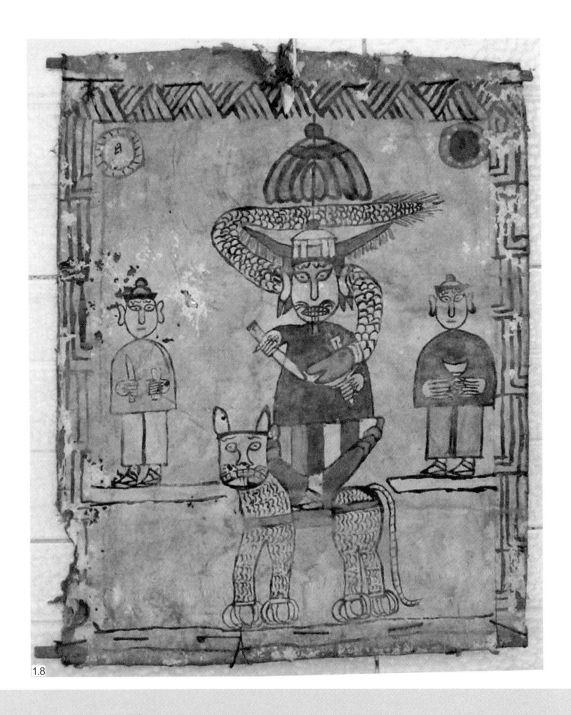

图 1.8

思茅疟疾暴发流行初期，巫师用于驱邪治病骗钱的神像。

Fig. 1.8

In the early stage of the malaria epidemic outbreak in Simao, the picture of gods used by shamans to ward off evil spirits and cure diseases to cheat money.

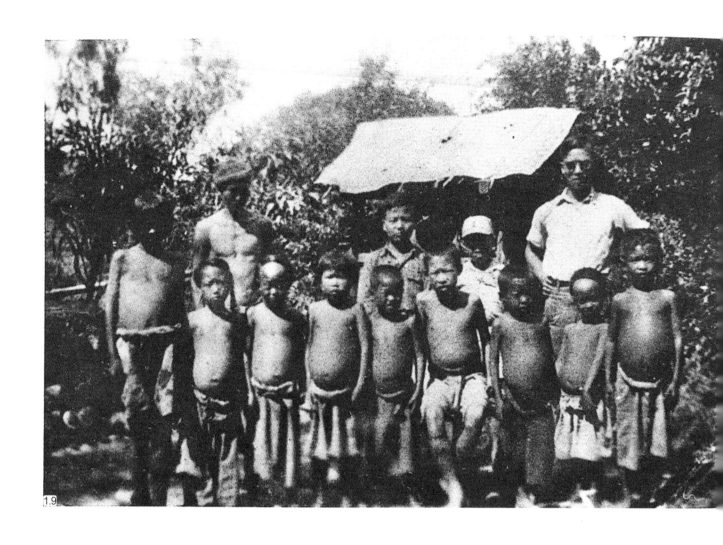

图 1.9~1.10
1940年郑祖佑医生在云县开展疟疾调查时，与因患疟疾脾肿大儿童合影。

Fig. 1.9-1.10
Two pictures of Dr. Zheng and the splenomegaly children due to malaria infection during his malaria investigation in 1940.

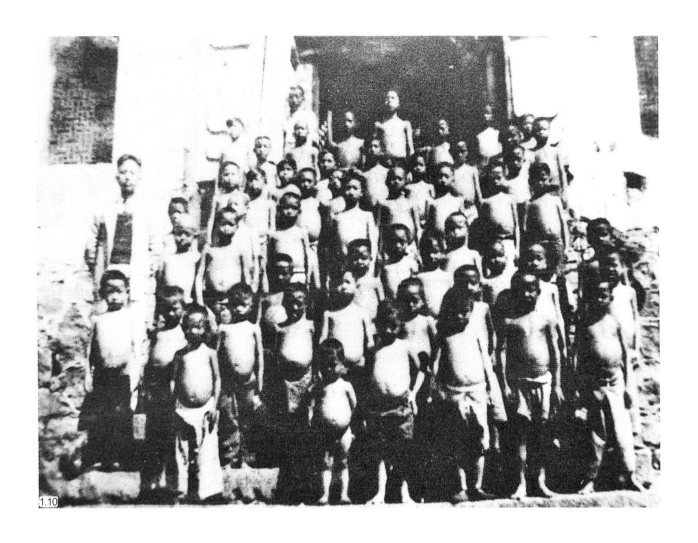

1944
1945
1946
1947
1948
1949
1950
1951
1952
1953
1954
1955
1956
1957
1958
1959
1960
1961
1962
1963
1964
1965
1966
1967
1968
1969
1970
1971
1972
1973
1974
1975
1976
1977
1978
1979
1980
1981
1982
1983
1984
1985
1986
1987
1988
1989
1990
1991
1992
1993
1994
1995
1996
1997
1998
1999
2000
2001
2002
2003
2004
2005
2006
2007
2008
2009
2010
2011
2012
2013
2014
2015
2016
2017
2018
2019
2020

1950

1955

1970

1985

2010

2020

Part 2
Malaria Baseline Survey and Pilot Control Program

1950—1955年属于云南省疟疾流行基线调查与防治试点阶段。滇南战役胜利后，1950年2月24日，中共云南省委正式成立，陈赓将军正式宣布云南完全解放。2000年1月17日，中共云南省委办公厅正式发文将1950年2月24日定为"云南解放日"。中国共产党本着"生命至上，健康至上"的原则，解放战争一结束，解放军就开始帮助地方政府开展疟疾防治工作。

1951年12月，经政务院文化教育委员会批准，印发《少数民族地区疟疾防治工作方案》，派遣中央防疫队、解放军防疫队、西南防疫队和云南省防疫队卫生专业人员进入云南少数民族聚居区，首先招募和培训当地的卫生人员，然后与当地卫生人员一起，边开展疟疾流行基线调查，边治疗病人和开展疟疾综合防治工作。

1952—1953年在全省129个县（市、区）中，抽样完成86个县（市）、199个区（乡、镇）的疟疾基线调查，结果显示均为疟疾流行区；1953年统计全省疟疾发病410 274人，发病率为249.38/万。基线调查获得了比较全面的云南疟疾流行资料。

1955年全国完成了疟疾流行基线调查，通过基线调查期间的疟疾防治工作，云南及其全国其他主要疟区的疟疾负担下降50%。1956年卫生部颁布了全国第一个疟疾防治五年规划，云南省也相应制定了云南省第一个疟疾防治五年规划。针对云南疟疾流行严重和媒介复杂的疟疾流行病学特征，通过防治试点，把全民服药根治、

图 2.1

解放军进入昆明，云南解放，至此云南开始了疟疾调查与防治工作。

Fig. 2.1

When the People's Liberation Army entered Kunming, Yunnan was liberated, and malaria investigation and prevention began.

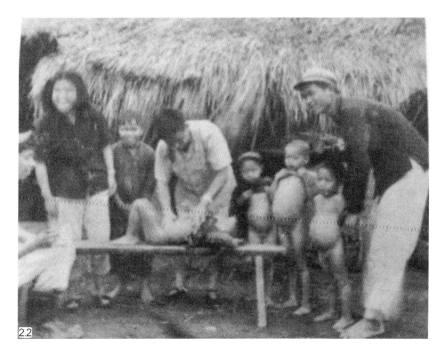

图 2.2

20世纪50年代，卫生人员深入村寨开展疟疾调查。图中为卫生人员检查儿童因疟疾感染引起的脾肿大。

Fig. 2.2

In the 1950s, health workers went into villages to investigate malaria. In the figure, health workers were examining the spleen in children.

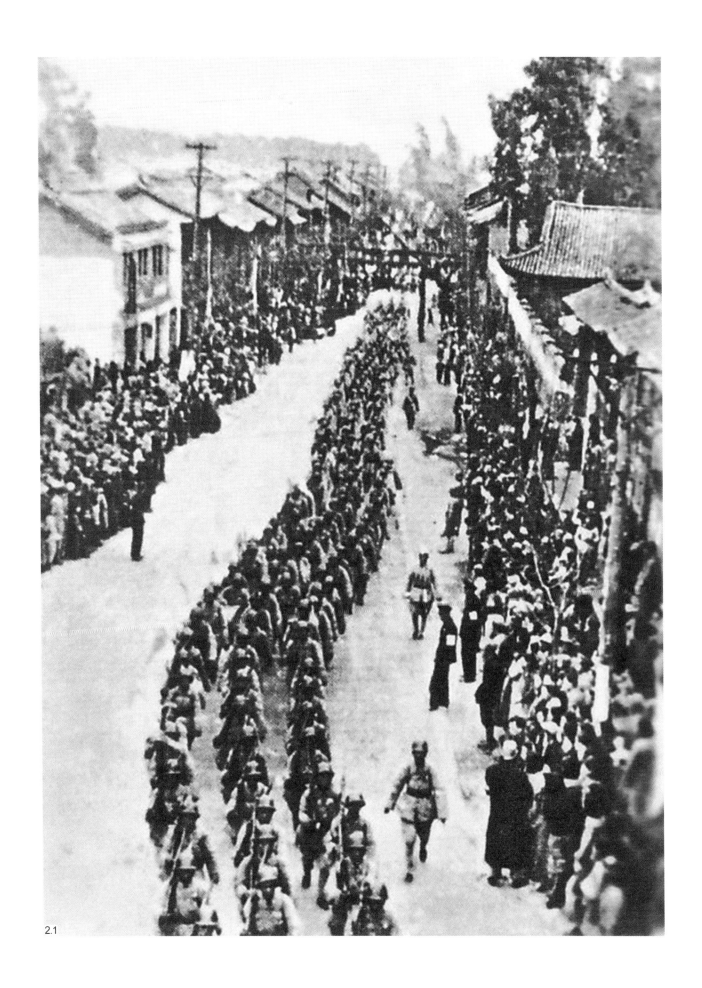

2.1

流行季节全民预防服药和全面杀虫剂室内滞留喷洒的"三全措施"作为云南疟疾防治主要策略。

The period from 1950 to 1955 was the phase of conducting baseline survey and pilot control program for malaria epidemic in Yunnan Province. After the victory of Southern Yunnan War, the Yunnan Provincial Committee of the Communist Party was formally established on 24 February, 1950 and General Chen Geng officially announced the complete liberation of Yunnan. The February 24th 1950 was officially designated as "Yunnan Liberation Day" in a document issued by the General Office of Yunnan Provincial Communist Party Committee. Based on the principle of "life first, health first", the Chinese Communist Party began to help the local government with malaria prevention and treatment activities as soon as the Liberation War ended.

In December 1951, the Culture and Education Committee of the Government Administration Council issued *The Work Protocol of Malaria Control in Ethnical Minority Areas*, and sent health professionals from the Central Antiepidemic Team, the Liberation Army Antiepidemic Team，the Southwestern Antiepidemic Team and Yunnan Antiepidemic Team, into hyperendemic areas of ethnical minority communities in Yunnan. Initially, these dispatched health professionals recruited and trained local health staff, and then they carried out a baseline epidemiological survey together, while treating malaria patients and carrying out integrated malaria control measures.

In Yunnan, the baseline malaria investigation was conducted in a sample of 199 townships, 86 counties out of 129 counties during 1952-1953. The results of baseline survey indicated that all of them were malaria endemic areas. In 1953 alone, there were 41 0274 malaria cases detected, and the malaria incidence rate was 24.938 per 1 000 person-years in the Province. The survey provided relatively comprehensive data on malaria prevalence in Yunnan Province.

By 1955, China had completed the baseline survey nationwide, and the control interventions reduced malaria burden by about 50% in main endemic areas including Yunnan and other major malaria-endemic regions of China. Outcomes and information gained from the baseline survey and the early control strategies helped the National Ministry of Health develop "The 1st National Malaria Control Plan for Five-Year" in 1956. Yunnan Province also formulated and then issued "Yunnan Provincial Control Plan for the 1st Five-Year". In response to the epidemiological characteristics with high malaria burden and complex vectors in Yunnan Province, "three comprehensive measures" for malaria control, i.e. mass drug distribution for radical cure, universal preventive treatment with available antimalarial drugs and full indoor residual spraying of insecticides in malaria transmitting seasons, were undertaken as the main strategies for malaria control in Yunnan Province.

图 2.3

某农村1951年检查出因疟疾感染脾肿大的儿童合影。

Fig. 2.3

A group picture of splenomegaly children due to malaria infection in a village in 1951.

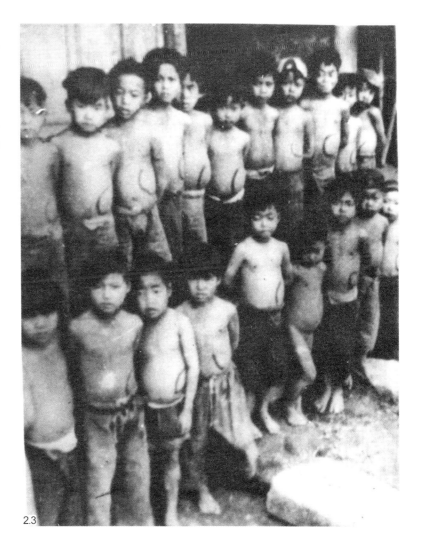

2.3

图 2.4

20世纪50年代，解放军卫生人员深入江城县哈尼族村寨为村民诊治疟疾。

Fig. 2.4

A health worker from the People's Liberation Army went into a Hani ethnic minority village in Jiangcheng County to diagnose and treat malaria for villagers in 1950s.

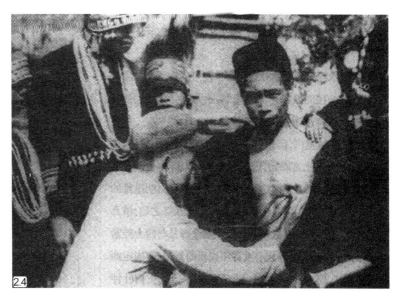

2.4

1944
1945
1946
1947
1948
1949
1950 — 1950
1951
1952
1953
1954
1955 — 1955
1956
1957
1958
1959
1960
1961
1962
1963
1964
1965
1966
1967
1968
1969
1970 — 1970
1971
1972
1973
1974
1975
1976
1977
1978
1979
1980
1981
1982
1983
1984
1985 — 1985
1986
1987
1988
1989
1990
1991
1992
1993
1994
1995
1996
1997
1998
1999
2000
2001
2002
2003
2004
2005
2006
2007
2008
2009
2010 — 2010
2011
2012
2013
2014
2015
2016
2017
2018
2019
2020 — 2020

第三部分
控制疟疾发病率

Part 3
Controlling the Incidence of Malaria

1956年，中央、西南和云南防疫队人员，在普洱县（今宁洱县）正式建立云南省第一疟疾防治所，1957年与1958年又先后在潞西县（今芒市）、耿马成立了云南省第二与第三疟疾防治所。云南其他地区的人员也相应成立了当地疟疾防治所或疟疾防治站。1957年在云南省第一疟疾防治所的基础上，在勐海县成立了云南省疟疾防治所，1968年该所从勐海搬迁到思茅，1984年更名为云南省疟疾防治研究所，2001云南省疾病预防控制体制改革，更名为云南省寄生虫病防治所。此外，云南省第二与第三疟疾防治所分别更名为潞西县卫生防疫站（现为芒市疾病预防控制中心）和耿马县卫生防疫站，其他地区疟疾防治所或疟疾防治站也更名为卫生防疫站。

1956—1970年为第一、第二和第三个疟疾防治五年规划执行期。三个五年规划的实施，全面降低了全省疟疾发病率。

第一个五年规划（1956—1960年）期间，继续在全省招募人员，开展疟疾防治知识和技术培训，进一步完善全省疟疾防治机构；同时在勐海县和梁河县开展疟疾防治（当时称消灭疟疾）试点，然后根据试点结果，制定了全省疟疾防治的策略与措施，推广了试点经验。第二个五年规划（1961—1965年）和第三个五年规划（1966—1970年）期间，首先根据流行程度把全省划分成疟疾高度流行区、中度流行区和低度流行区。在高度流行区继续使用"三全措施"降低疟疾发病率。中、低度流行区以控制传染源为主，及时规范治疗现症病人和带虫者，对有疟疾发病史者进行休止期根治；根据媒介监测结果，对重点村寨开展杀虫剂室内滞留喷洒；对前往高流行区重点人员（例如河谷地区下坝生产人员）开展预防服药。

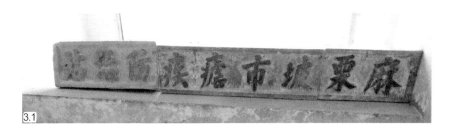

3.1

图 3.1
1957年成立的麻栗坡市疟疾防治站的匾牌（后更名为麻栗坡县防疫站，现名麻栗坡县疾控中心）。

Fig. 3.1
The plaque of Malipo City Station for Malaria Control founded in 1957, （renamed as Malipo County Antiepidemic Station later, Malipo County Center for Disease Control at present）.

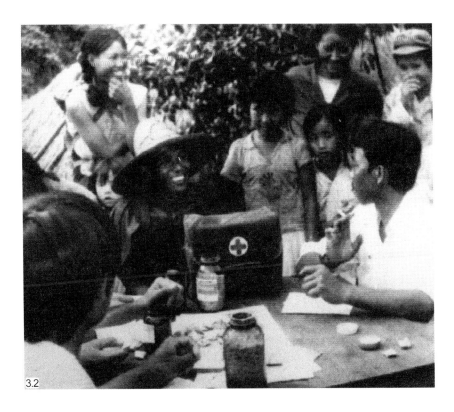

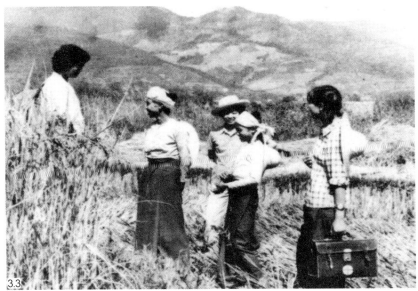

图 3.2~3.3

20世纪50年代至60年代，卫生人员深入山村、田间为群众诊治疟疾。

Fig. 3.2-3.3

The health workers went into remote villages and fields to diagnose and treat malaria for villagers in 1950s and 1960s.

到1960年，全省建立了功能完备的疟疾防治卫生服务体系。如1957年5月开始的勐海坝试点，到1962年底已实现无当地新感染疟疾病例，达到了当时卫生部颁布的基本消灭疟疾标准。第一个五年规划期间全省报告疟疾病人644 179例，年平均128 836例，较防治前（1952—1955年）的年平均312 779例下降了58.81%。第二和第三个五年规划进一步完善县、乡、村三级疟疾防护网，健全了基层卫生组织，开展疟疾健康教育，发动群众参与疟疾防治工作。到1970年全省疟疾发病率控制到了24.32/万，低于全国29.61/万的疟疾发病率。

In 1956, the personnel from the Central Antiepidemic Team, the Southwestern Antiepidemic Team and Yunnan Antiepidemic Team established the first Yunnan Institute of Malaria Control (YIMC) in Pu'er (Ning'er, currently) County. In 1957, the second YIMC was established in Luxi (Mangshi, currently), and in 1958 the third YIMC was established in Gengma. In other parts of Yunnan, the local institutes or stations for malaria control were also set up. Yunnan Institute of Malaria Control was founded in Menghai County on the basis of the first YIMC, which was removed to Simao in 1968 and then renamed as Yunnan Research Institute for Malaria Control (YRIMC) again in 1984. As a result of the systemic reform for disease control and prevention system in Yunnan，the YRIMC was renamed as Yunnan Institute of Parasitic Diseases in 2001. In addition, the second and third YIMC were renamed as Luxi Antiepidemic Station (Mangshi Centre for Disease Control and Preven-

图 3.4

20世纪70年代，卫生人员深入到田间对群众开展面对面的疟疾健康教育。

Fig. 3.4

The health workers carried out face-to-face health education about malaria in fields in the 1970s.

图 3.5

20世纪60年代，景谷县防疫站疟防人员深入村寨农户开展疟疾病例主动侦察（采血）。

Fig. 3.5

The healthcare staff from the Jinggu Antiepidemic Station was preparing blood collecting during their active malaria surveillance for fieldworkers of a remote village in the 1960s.

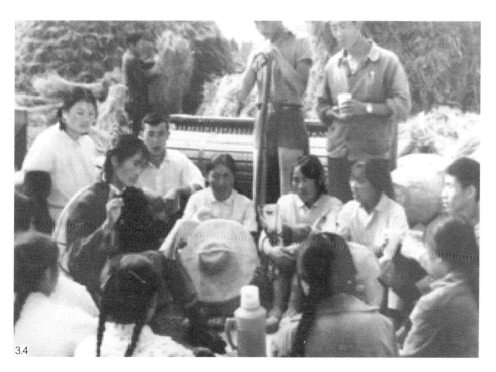

3.4

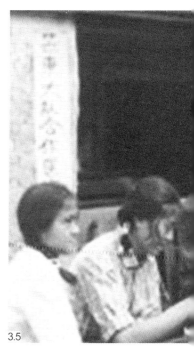

3.5

图 3.6

20世纪60年代至70年代,卫生人员深入傣族村寨为傣族居民诊治疟疾。

Fig. 3.6

The health workers went into Dai villages to diagnose and treat malaria for the Dai people in the 1950s and 1960s.

图 3.7

20世纪60年代至70年代,卫生人员深入村寨开展疟原虫带虫率调查（采血）。

Fig. 3.7

The health workers were collecting blood samples during an investigation of Plasmodium parasite rate in villages in the 1960s and 1970s.

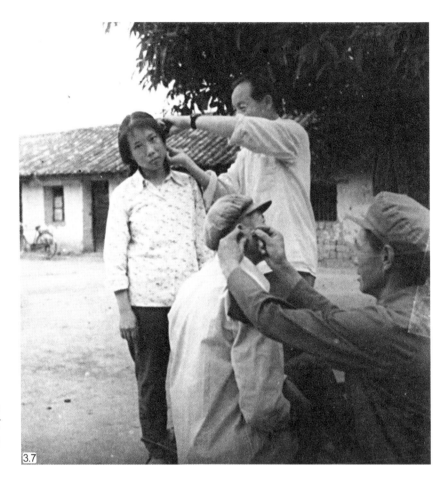

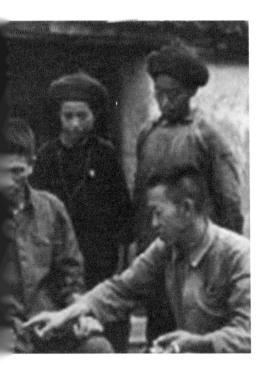

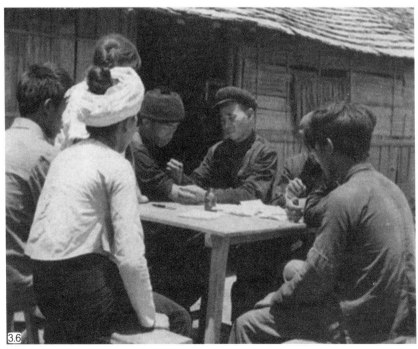

tion at present) and Gengma Antiepidemic Station, and those institutes or stations of malaria control in other regions were also renamed as the local antiepidemic stations later, respectively.

The years 1956-1970 was the implementation phase of the 1st, the 2nd and the 3rd Five-Year Plan for Malaria Control. The implementation significantly reduced the incidence of malaria across the Province.

During the 1st Five-Year Plan (1956-1960), the Province continued recruiting and training personnel on malaria control knowledge and skills, and further improved the health system for malaria prevention and control. At the same time, the Province carried out pilot malaria control (called as Malaria Eradication at that time) in Menghai and Lianghe Counties. Based on the pilot results the Province developed its strategies and measures for malaria control, and spread the pilot experience. During the 2nd Five-Year Plan (1961-1965) and the 3rd Five-Year Plan (1966-1970), the whole province was firstly divided into high, moderate and low malaria endemic areas based on malaria burden. The "three comprehensive measures" continued to be conducted to reduce malaria incidence in the high malaria endemic areas. In the moderate and low malaria endemic areas, the strategy focused on controlling the source of infection, and was to provide timely standardized treatment to clinical patients and parasite carriers in time, and radical treatment to those with a history of malaria infection in low malaria transmitting season. Drawing on results of vectors surveillance, the indoor residual spraying with insecticides was carried out in potential transmitting villages, and preventive treatment was delivered to the personnel traveling to high endemic areas, for example, people who went for agriculture

图 3.8~3.9

20世纪60年代至70年代，卫生人员送药到各村寨开展疟疾预防服药活动。

Fig. 3.8-3.9

The health workers went to the villages to deliver anti-malarial drugs for malaria preventive treatment in the 1960s and 1970s.

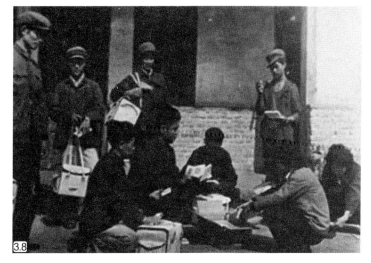

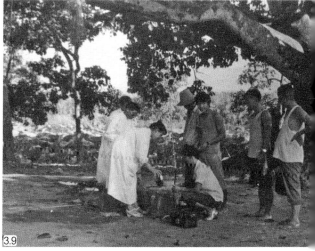

图 3.10

20世纪70年代，卫生人员深入村寨进行疟疾休止期根治，做到"送药送水到手，看服到口，咽下才走"。

Fig. 3.10

The health workers went to the remote villages to conduct radical treatment for malaria in a family house in the 1970s. They followed the request of "Distribute drugs and water to the individual's hand, watch him finish taking, and do not leave until the drugs are swallowed".

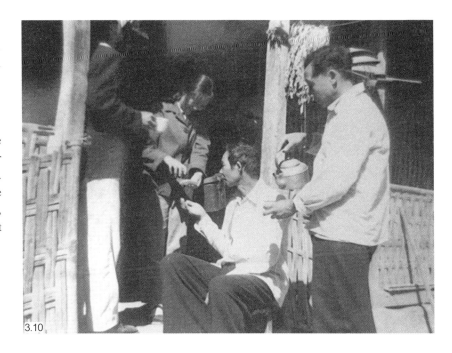

图 3.11~3.12

20世纪60年代至70年代，疟疾防治人员在人房和牛房开展传疟媒介按蚊人工小时密度调查。

Fig. 3.11-3.12

In the 1960s and 1970s, health workers conducted manual hourly density investigation of the malaria vector Anopheline mosquitoes in houses and cowsheds.

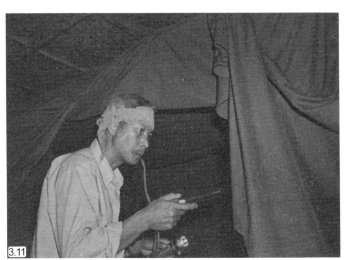

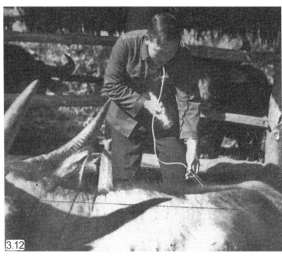

production in river valley areas.

By 1960, Yunnan had established a fully functional health system for malaria control. The pilot malaria control program that started in Menghai County in May 1957 achieved zero indigenous malaria case by the end of 1962, meeting the standard for the basic elimination of malaria issued by the Ministry of Health. During the 1st Five-Year Plan period 644 179 cases of malaria were reported in the whole province, with an annual average of 128 836 cases, which was 58.81% lower than the annual average of 312 779 cases before the prevention and treatment (1952-1955). The 2nd and 3rd Five-Year Plans further improved the malaria control networks at county, township and village levels, improved grass-roots health organizations, conducted health education, and mobilized the public to participate in malaria control. By 1970, the malaria incidence rate in the Province was reduced to 2.432 per 1 000 person-years, which was lower than the national malaria incidence rate 2.961 per 1 000 person-years across China.

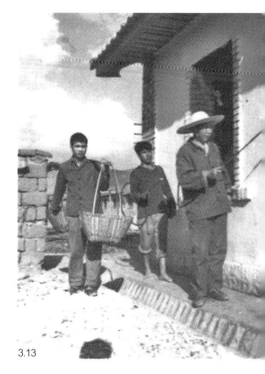

3.13

图 3.13

20世纪70年代，村寨组织开展杀虫剂滞留喷洒灭蚊工作。

Fig. 3.13

In the 1970s, villagers were carrying out residual spraying with insecticides to kill mosquitoes.

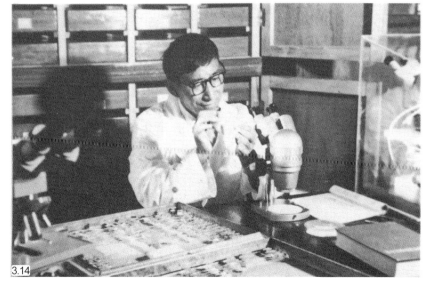

3.14

图 3.14

20世纪70年代，著名蚊虫专家董学书先生在做蚊虫分类鉴定。

Fig. 3.14

Mr. Dong Xueshu, a famous mosquito expert, was identifying mosquitoes in the 1970s.

图 3.15~3.16

20世纪50年代至60年代，各级举办了大量各类培训班，培训疟疾防治专业技术人员。右图：1963年全省疟疾培训班西双版纳景洪县六区（现大渡岗乡和基诺乡等地）实习组师生合影；下图：1964年思茅专区（现普洱市）疟疾培训班师生合影。

Fig. 3.15-3.16

In the 1950s and 1960s, a large number of training courses were held at each level to train malaria control professionals. Right Fig.: The group photo of teachers and students who participated in the Provincial Malaria Training Workshop in the sixth district (Dadugang and Ji'nuo Townships, etc., at present) of Jinghong County, Xishuangbanna in 1963. Fig. below: the photo of teachers and students of malaria training class in the Simao Prefecture (Pu'er Municipality at present) in 1964.

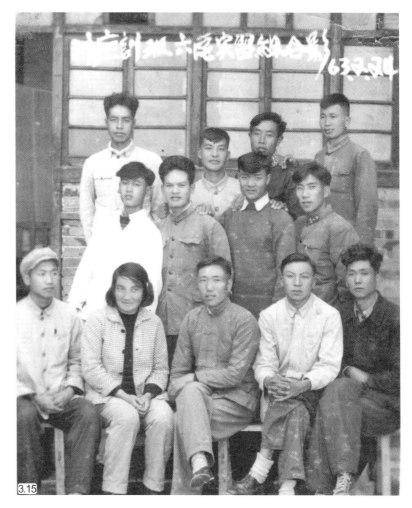

3.15

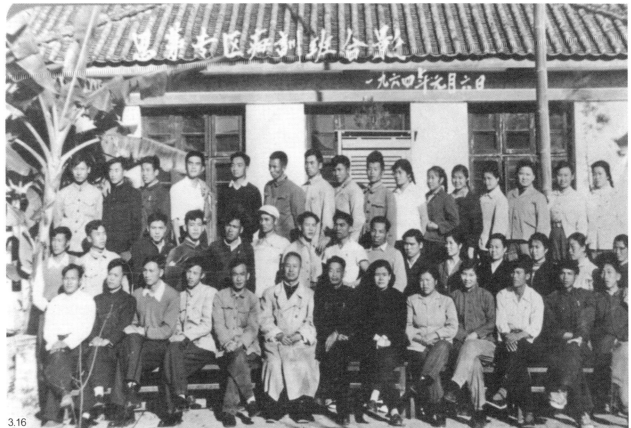

3.16

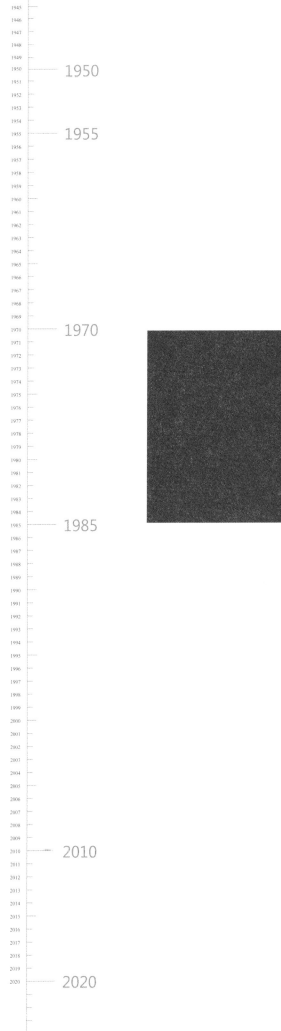

1950

1955

1970

1985

2010

2020

第四部分
疟疾大幅回升与控制暴发流行

Part 4
Malaria Resurgence and Outbreak Control

1971—1985年是云南省疟疾大幅回升与控制暴发流行阶段。受"文化大革命"的影响，部分防疫机构被解散，疟疾防治措施不能有效贯彻落实，同时人员流动大，疟疾扩散加快。1968年全省疟疾疫情开始反弹，1969年首先在保山市昌宁县湾甸公社热水社出现点状暴发流行，1971年盈江县和龙陵县出现片状大面积暴发流行，1973年疟疾流行程度达到最高峰，全省各地均有不同程度的点片暴发，疟疾发病154 384人，发病率高达56.18/万，是1970年24.32/万的2.3倍。

为控制疟疾暴发流行，1971年在盈江县旧城公社贺勐大队设置暴发控制试点，防疫人员入村驻队，强化了"全面杀虫剂室内滞留喷洒、全民预防服药和全民休止期根治"的"三全措施"，做到"送药到手，看服下肚，不吃不走"。根据试点经验，制定了云南省控制疟疾暴发流行技术方案，并在全省推广应用，采取重点地区重点防治、重点人群重点保护的分类防治策略，扑灭了疟疾暴发流行的苗头，扭转了疟疾回升势头。第四个疟疾防治五年规划

图4.1

云南1971年总结盈江疟疾暴发控制试点工作经验，制定了云南省控制疟疾暴发流行技术方案，并在盈江现场举办全省疟疾防治工作学习班推广。

Fig. 4.1

Based on the experiences of pilot malaria control in Yingjiang, *the Technical Protocol for Malaria Outbreak Control in Yunnan Province* was formulated. A training course for malaria control work was held in Yingjiang to publicize the experiences across the whole province in 1971.

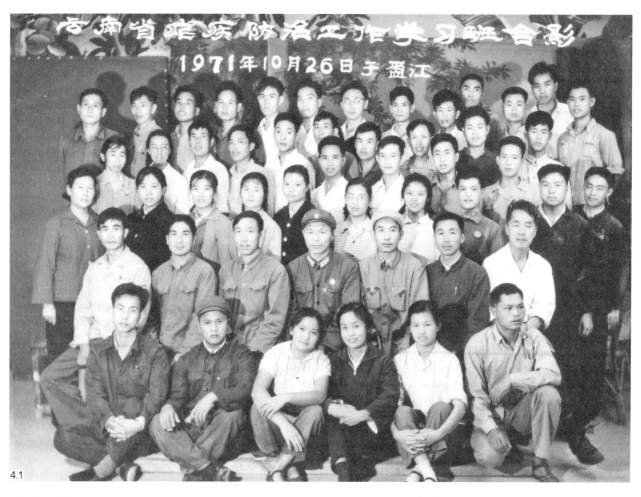

4.1

图 4.2

1971年盈江县大面积疟疾暴发流行，保山抗疟支队支援盈江县，控制疟疾暴发。

Fig. 4.2

During the epidemic of malaria in Yingjiang County in 1971, an expert team of Baoshan Municipality went down to Yingjiang County to support malaria outbreak control.

图 4.3

1974年云南省疟疾发病达到最高峰，为控制疟疾暴发流行，云南省疟疾训练班卫生人员培训后随即奔赴抗疟前线。

Fig. 4.3

In 1974, malaria morbidity rebounded to the peak in Yunnan Province. In order to control the outbreak, health workers immediately went to fields to fight malaria outbreaks after training.

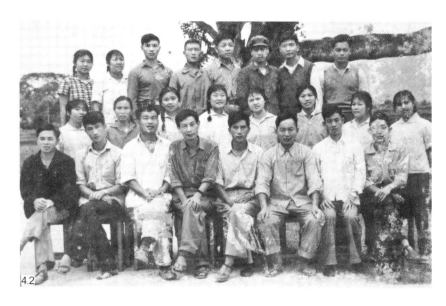

4.2

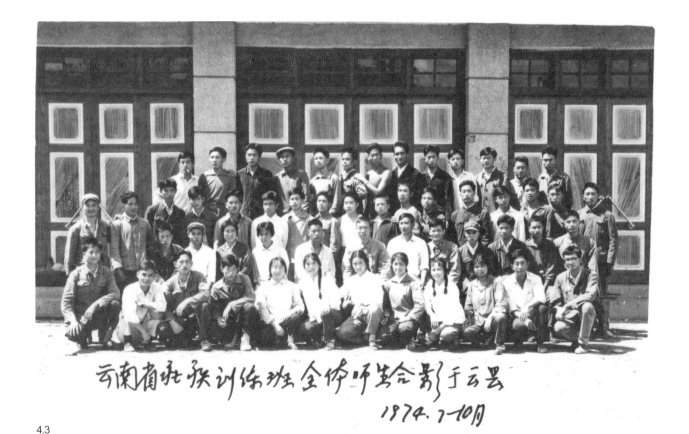

4.3

（1971—1975年）末期，疟疾迅猛回升的势头得到有效遏制。第五个五年规划（1976—1980年）和第六个五年规划（1981—1985年）期间，疟疾逐渐得到有效控制，全省发病数从"四五"规划的550 416例下降至"五五"规划的189 599例；年平均发病数从110 083例下降到37 920例，下降了65.56%；年平均发病率从40.14/万下降至12.31/万，下降了69.33%。"六五"规划与"五五"规划相比，年平均发病数下降38.34%，年平均发病率下降42.00%。1985年全省疟疾发病率下降到5.67/万。

图 4.7~4.8
20世纪70年代，入村驻队人员在村社开展疟疾防治知识宣传。

Fig. 4.7-4.8
In the 1970s, healthcare workers stationed in villages conducted health education on malaria.

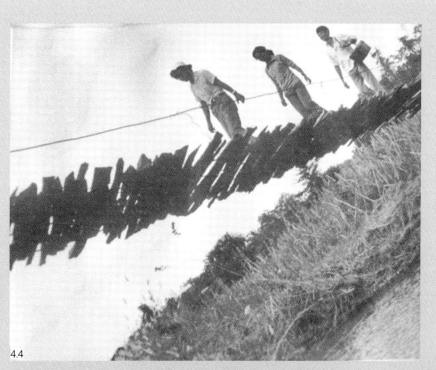

4.4

图 4.4~4.6
20世纪70年代，疟防人员跋山涉水，挥洒青春热血和汗水，深入村寨开展疟疾防治工作。

Fig. 4.4-4.6
Healthcare workers climbed hills and forded streams to sprinkle the blood and sweat of youth to deliver malaria control services to villages in the 1970s.

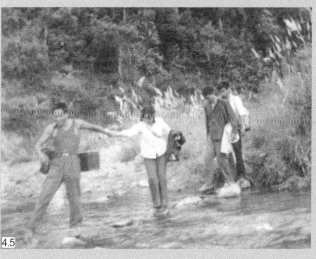

4.5

4.6

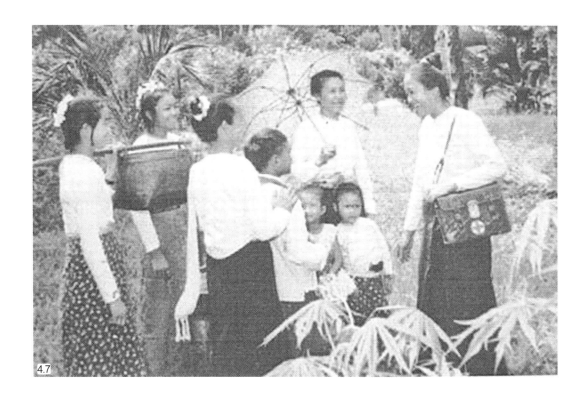

4.7

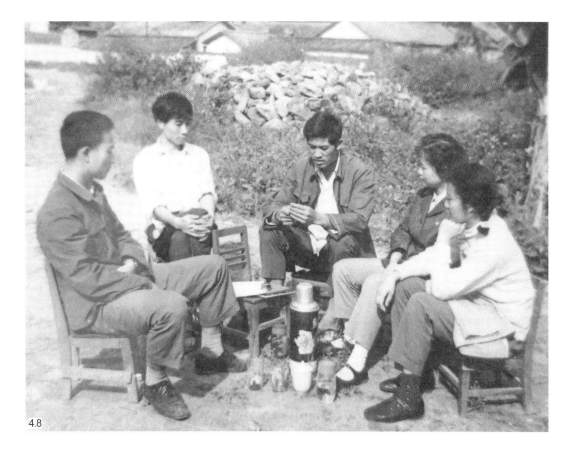

4.8

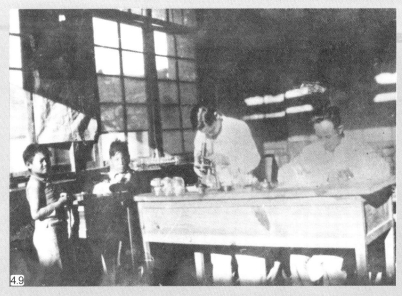

4.9

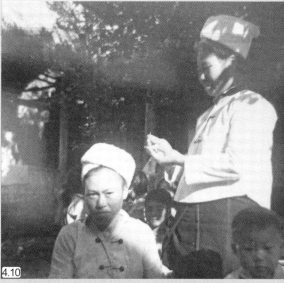

4.10

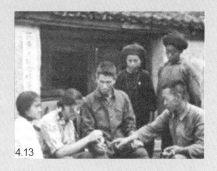

4.13

Years 1971-1985 was the phase of malaria resurgence and outbreak control for Yunnan. The malaria epidemic in the whole province began to gradually rebound in 1968 under the influence of "the Great Cultural Revolution" that disbanded the anti-epidemic stations and the slow the progress of some malaria control measures, as well as the high mobility of people accelerated the spread. The first outbreak occurred in Reshui Village of Wandian Commune, Changning County, Baoshan Municipality in 1969. Two epidemics occurred in Yingjiang County and Longling County respectively in 1971. Malaria prevalence rebounded to its peak in the provincewide epidemic in 1973, with a total of 154 384 malaria cases and the annual malaria incidence (AMI) reached 5.618 per 1 000 person-years reported. The AMI was 2.3 times of AMI 2.432 per 1 000 person-years in 1970.

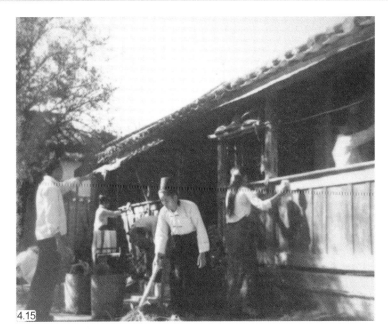

4.15

图 4.15

20世纪70年代，抗疟人员入村驻队动员村民开展爱国卫生运动灭蚊活动。

Fig. 4.15

In the 1970s, healthcare workers stationed in villages mobilized villagers carrying out the patriotic health campaign to repell mosquitoes in villages.

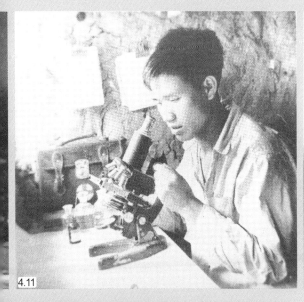

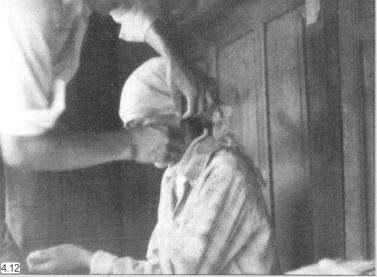

图 4.9~4.14

20世纪70年代，抗疟人员入村驻队开展全民疟原虫血检工作。

Fig. 4.9-4.14

In the 1970s, healthcare workers stationed in villages carried out the blood examination for malaria parasites for all residents in villages.

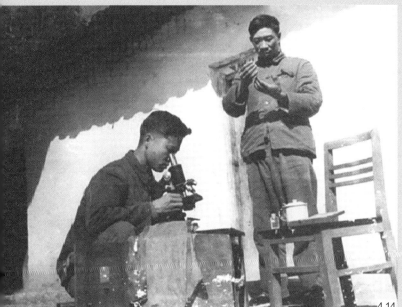

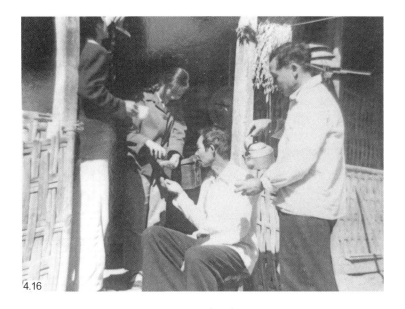

图 4.16

20世纪70年代，抗疟人员入村驻队开展全民服药，做到"送药到手，看服下肚，不吃不走"。

Fig. 4.16

In the 1970s, healthcare workers stationed in villages conducted mass drug distribution for malaria preventive and radical treatment by the house-to-house visits daily to deliver drugs and conduct directly observed therapy.

In order to control the epidemic, a pilot intervention program was carried out in Hemeng Village of Jiucheng Commune, Yingjiang County in 1971. Healthcare workers were stationed in villages to strengthen the "three comprehensive measures" i.e. full indoor residual spraying with insecticides, mass drug distribution for preventive treatments and radical cure treatment, respectively. In order to achieve the goal, the universal actions requested health workers to execute house-to-house visits every day to deliver drugs and conduct directly observed therapy. According to the experience of the pilot trial, *a Technical Protocol of Outbreak Control* was formulated and applied in the whole province. The epidemic and increasing incidence trend was effectively reversed by using strategies like key interventions for the key areas, the key protection for the populations at the high risk. As a results of implementation of outbreak control, the rapidly increasing malaria prevalence was halted by the end of the 4th Five-Year Plan for Malaria Control (FYPMC) 1971-1975. Malaria morbidity was gradually reduced in the 5th (1976-1980) and 6th (1980-1985) FYPMC period. The number of cases in the Province dropped from a total of 550 416 in the 4th FYPMC to a total of 189 599 in the 5th FYPMC. The average annual cases achieved 65.56% decrease, reduced from a total of 110 083 to 37 920. The AMI dropped by 69.33%, from 4.014 per 1 000 person-years to 1.231 per 1 000 person-years. The number of average annual cases in the 6th FYPMC was decreased by 38.34%, and the AMI decreased by 42% in comparison with the 5th FYPMC. By 1985, the AMI decreased to 0.567 per 1 000 person-years.

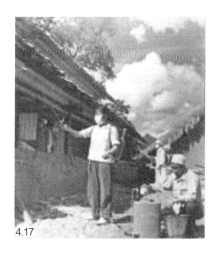

4.17

图 4.17~4.19

20世纪70年代，抗疟人员入村驻队组织开展全面杀虫剂室内滞留喷洒工作。

Fig. 4.17-4.19

In the 1970s, healthcare workers stationed in villages carried out universal indoor residual spraying with insecticides in villages.

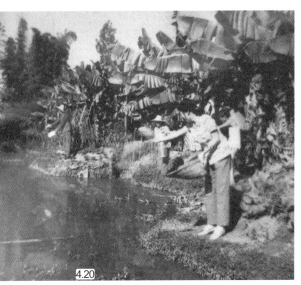

4.20

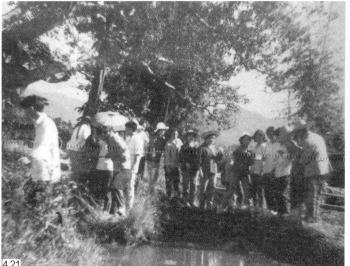

4.21

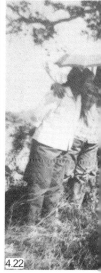

4.22

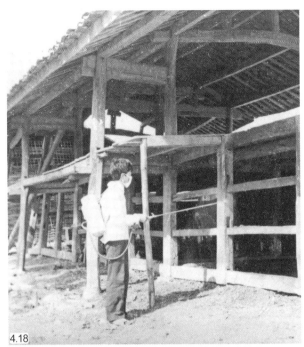

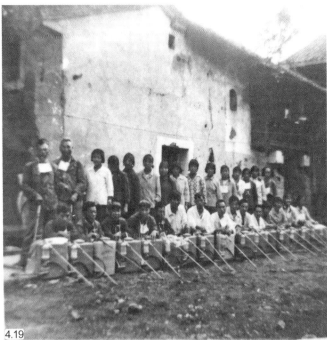

图 **4.20~4.24**

20世纪70年代，抗疟人员入村驻队开展媒介滋生地调查与处置工作。

Fig. 4.20-4.24

In the 1970s, healthcare workers stationing villages investigated and disposes vector breeding sites in the field.

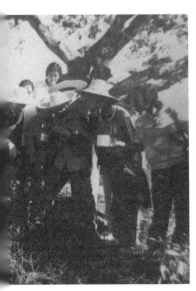

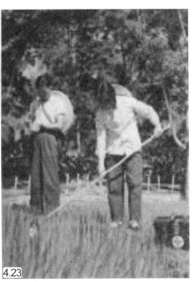

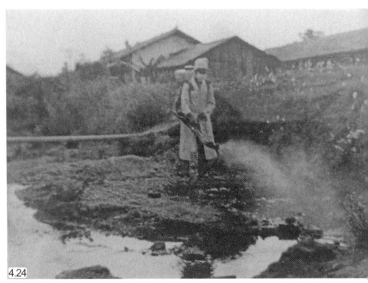

1944
1945
1946
1947
1948
1949
1950   1950
1951
1952
1953
1954
1955   1955
1956
1957
1958
1959
1960
1961
1962
1963
1964
1965
1966
1967
1968
1969
1970   1970
1971
1972
1973
1974
1975
1976
1977
1978
1979
1980
1981
1982
1983
1984
1985   1985
1986
1987
1988
1989
1990
1991
1992
1993
1994
1995
1996
1997
1998
1999
2000
2001
2002
2003
2004
2005
2006
2007
2008
2009
2010   2010
2011
2012
2013
2014
2015
2016
2017
2018
2019
2020   2020

第五部分
降低发病率和巩固扩大防治成果

Part 5
Consolidating and Scaling Up Achievement

1986—2010年是降低发病率和巩固扩大防治成果阶段。随着国民经济持续增长，疟疾防治工作得到逐步加强，进一步夯实了"重点地区重点防治、重点人群重点保护、因地制宜分类防治"策略和措施。特别是20世纪90年代初中期拟除虫菊酯类新型杀虫剂和青蒿素类等高效抗疟药的推广应用，提高了防治效果。1986—2000年执行第七、第八、第九个疟疾防治五年规划期间，全省疟疾发病率稳步下降，疟疾得到较好的控制。全省发病数从"七五"规划（1986—1990年）的82 118例下降至"九五"规划（1996—2000年）的59 910例；年平均发病数从16 423例下降到11 982例，下降了27.04%；年平均发病率从4.62/万下降至3.02/万，下降了34.63%；2000年全省疟疾发病率下降至2.23/万。但由于热区农业开发和边境贸易的深入发展，人口流动频繁，疟疾输入病例（含跨境输入）剧增，边境25县（市）和元江流域在"八五"规划期间出现疟疾点状暴发，"九五"规划期间疟疾发病数占全省发病数的70%以上，成为疟疾流行程度高、控制难度大的地区。

2000年前后，云南疟疾防治逐步与国际接轨，2001年加入WHO湄公河遏制疟疾规划项目，获得经费人民币210万元。2003—2010年，云南省获得全球基金抗击艾滋病、结核病和疟疾项目第一、第五和第六轮资助，累计获得近1.8亿元人民币和物资支持，全省74个疟疾重点县的防治能力得到进一步加强，防治工作得到规范

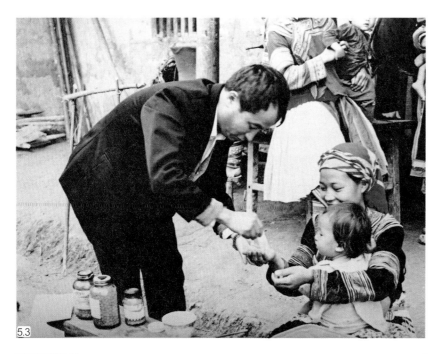

5.3

图 5.1~5.5

20世纪80年代至90年代，采取"重点
地区重点防治、重点人群重点保护、
因地制宜分类防治"策略，抗疟人员
深入重点村寨开展全民服药工作。

Fig. 5.1-5.5

In the 1980s and 1990s, healthcare personnel conducted mass drug distribution in villages based on the strategy of "local oriented, burden oriented, special strategy for special area".

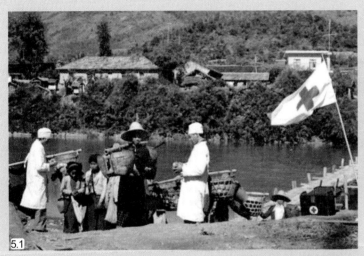

5.1

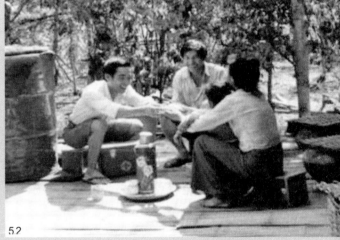

5.2

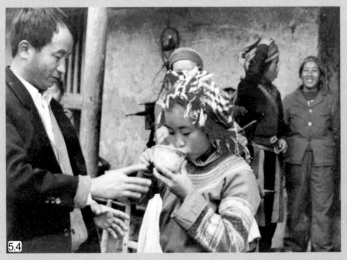

5.4

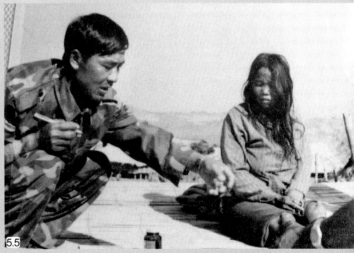

5.5

化管理，特别是边境25县（市）建立了跨境联防联控合作机制，重点实施以境外80个疟疾诊治站和境内68个疟疾咨询服务站为主的边境疟疾三道防线策略，境外疟疾流行程度得到有效遏制，境内防治成果得到巩固扩大，全省发病率持续下降。本地感染病例逐年减少，全省发病数从"十五"规划（2001—2005年）的62 804例下降至"十一五"规划（2006—2010年）的29 756例；年平均发病数从12 560例下降到5 951例，下降了52.62%；年平均发病率从2.98/万下降至1.26/万，下降了57.77%；2010年全省疟疾发病率下降至0.48/万，仅17个中缅边境县（市）有本地感染疟疾病例和发病率大于1/万。

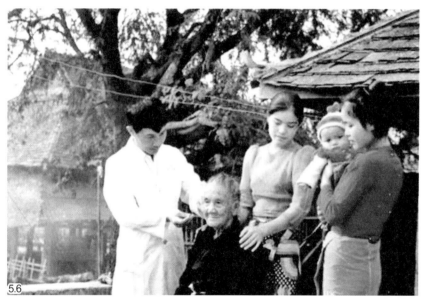

5.6

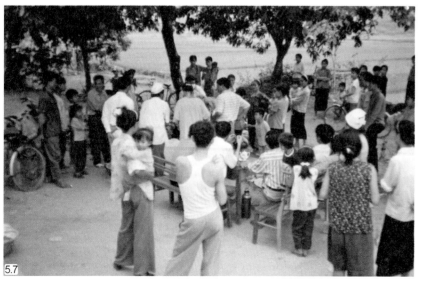

5.7

图 5.6~5.7
20世纪80年代至90年代，抗疟人员深入重点村寨开展全民血检筛查疟原虫。

Fig. 5.6-5.7

In the 1980s and 1990s, healthcare personnel conducted blood examination to screen malaria in endemic villages.

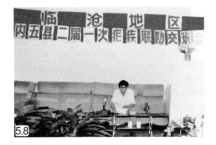

5.8

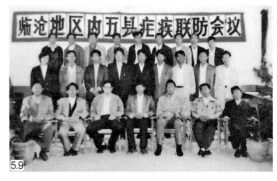

5.9

图 5.8~5.9

20世纪90年代，以州（市）为单位开展区域内疟疾联防联控，每年由值班县召开年会，交流防治经验。

Fig. 5.8-5.9

In the 1990s, the joint prevention and control of malaria was established at prefecture (city) level, and the counties on duty convened the annual meeting every year to summarize and exchange the control experience.

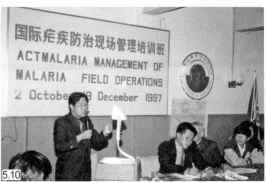

5.10

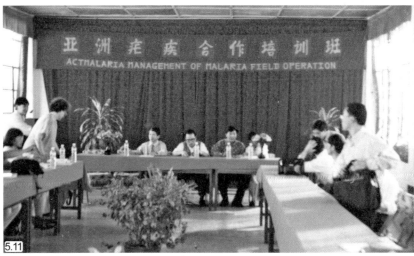

5.11

图 5.10~5.12

20世纪90年代中后期，云南疟疾防治逐渐与国际接轨，1997年与泰国合作，在泰国和云南举办首届亚洲疟疾培训网络（ACT）疟疾防治现场管理国际培训班；1997年ACT资助在思茅市（今普洱市）举办全国疟疾防治现场管理培训班。

Fig. 5.10-5.12

Malaria control in Yunnan was gradually connecting with international organizations in the middle and late 1990s. Collaborating with Thailand, the first training course on management of malaria field operation funded by Asian Collaborative Training Network for Malaria (ACT Malaria) was hold in Thailand and Yunnan, respectively in 1997. ACT Malaria supported and funded Yunnan to hold the national training course on management of malaria field operation for Chinese participants in 1997.

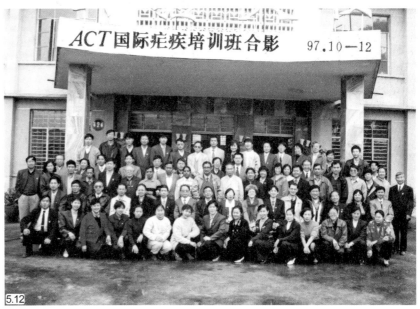

5.12

The period 1986-2010 was the phase of rolling back malaria to consolidate and scale up control achievement. The work of fighting malaria has been further strengthened with the continuous growth of the national economy. The strategies and measures of "local oriented, burden oriented, special strategy for special area" have been strengthened, the achievement further consolidated. Especially in the early and middle 1990s, the application of new pyrethroid insecticides and artemisinins and other highly effective antimalarial drugs improved the control effect. During the implementation of the 7th, 8th and 9th FYPMC from 1986 to 2000, malaria morbidity in the Province had been steadily declining and malaria epidemic had been well controlled. The number of malaria cases dropped from a total of 82 118 in the 7th FYPMC (1986-1990) to a total of 59 910 in the 9th FYPMC (1996-2000). The annual average number of cases decreased from 16 423 to 11 982, down by 27.04%, and AMI dropped by 34.63%, from 0.462 per 1 000 person-years to 0.302 per 1 000 person-years. However, due to the development of agriculture in the tropical areas and further development of border trade, increased population movement led to sharp rise of imported cases (including cross-border importation). The 25 border counties (cities) and Yuanjiang river basins became the areas of serious malaria prevalence with great difficulty in control. Malaria spot outbreaks frequently occurred during the 8th FYPMC (1991-1995), and the number of malaria cases accounted for more than 70% of the total cases of all diseases in the Province during the 9th FYPMC.

Malaria control in Yunnan was gradually in line with international standards around the turn of millennium. In Yunnan, the first inter-

图 5.13

2001年加入世界卫生组织湄公河遏制疟疾规划项目，项目周期为3年，项目经费人民币210万，主要内容是边境疟疾控制和恶性疟抗药性监测。

Fig. 5.13

In 2001, the World health Organization granted Yunnan the 3-year program of Roll Back Malaria in Mekong River Region with a budget of RMB 2.1 million. The goal was to roll back malaria and drug resistance surveillance of *Plasmodium falciparum* along the international border.

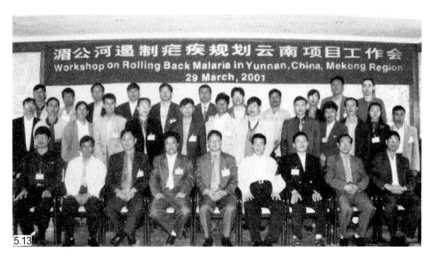

5.13

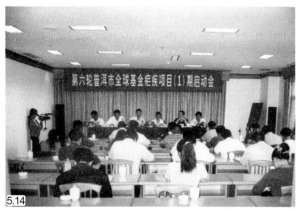

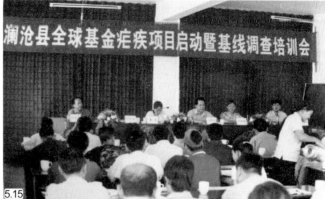

图 5.14~5.16

云南2003—2010年获得全球基金第一、第五和第六轮疟疾项目资助，云南74个疟疾重点县（市）的防治能力得到进一步加强，防治工作得到规范化管理。

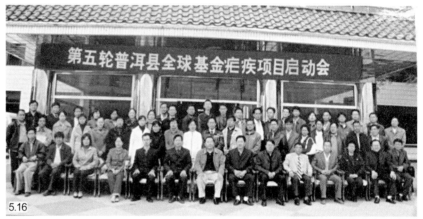

Fig. 5.14-5.16

Yunnan was granted by the first, fifth and sixth round of China GFATM malaria control projects from 2003 to 2010. The GFATM projects further strengthened the control capacities in 74 key counties (cities), and gradually standardized the management in malaria control.

图 5.17

自2000年以后，境外输入性疟疾严重威胁云南疟疾防治成果，在原国家卫生部和全球基金疟疾项目的支持下，云南与缅甸建立了边境地区疟疾联防联控合作，2005年举办中缅边境地区镜检技术培训班。

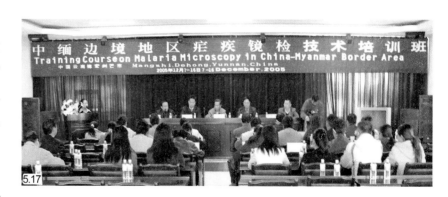

Fig. 5.17

After 2000, imported malaria seriously threatened the achievements of malaria control in Yunnan. With the supports of National Ministry of Health and the GFATM malaria projects, Yunnan and Myanmar established solid cooperation on joint prevention and control of malaria along the international border. An international training course on microscopy was held for the participants from China-Myanmar border areas in 2005.

national project was WHO Mekong Malaria Control Program that the WHO funded Yunnan with 2.1 million RMB in 2001. From 2003 to 2010, Yunnan won the first, fifth and sixth rounds of China malarial project of the Global Fund to Fight AIDS, Tuberculosis and Malaria (GFATM) with nearly RMB 180 million including budget of material support. By GFATM malaria projects, the prevention and control capacity of 74 counties (cities) where malaria was more serious than other parts in the province had been further strengthened and their management of malaria control was gradually standardized. Meanwhile, a joint cooperation mechanism and three preventive lines of cross-border malaria control had been established in 25 border counties (cities), in which 80 stations for malaria diagnosis and treatment were established in Myanmar and 68 border malaria consultation posts set up along the border in China. Great achievements have been made from the GFATM projects that malaria epidemic and incidence in Myanmar border areas had been effectively rolled back. The control achievements had been consolidated and scaled up in Yunnan. The malaria endemic areas were gradually shrunk, and the malaria morbidity continuously declined. As a result, the number of cases dropped from a total of 62 804 in the 10th FYPMC (2001-2005) to 29 756 in the 11th FYPMC (2006-2010). The annual average number of cases decreased from 12 560 to 5 951, down by 52.62%, and the AMI dropped by 57.77%, from 0.298 per 1 000 person-years to 0.126 per 1 000 person-years. By 2010, the malaria incidence in the Province decreased to 0.048 per 1 000 person-years. Only 17 China-Myanmar border counties (cities) had indigenous malaria cases, and were featured with an incidence greater than 0.1 per 1 000 person-years.

图 5.18~5.20

第一轮全球基金疟疾项目2003年对25个边境项目县（市）开展入户带虫率、漏报率和疟疾知识知晓率基线调查，调查结果为全省疟疾漏报率88.8%（27 155/30 580），初步摸清了云南边境地区疟疾流行态势。

Fig. 5.18-5.20

In 2003, the baseline survey on malaria parasite prevalence, underreported cases and knowledge was carried out with support of the first round of GFATM malaria project in 25 border counties (cities). The results showed that the underreported rate of malaria cases was 88.8% (27 155 / 30 580) in Yunnan, which made the true malaria situation clear in the border area of Yunnan.

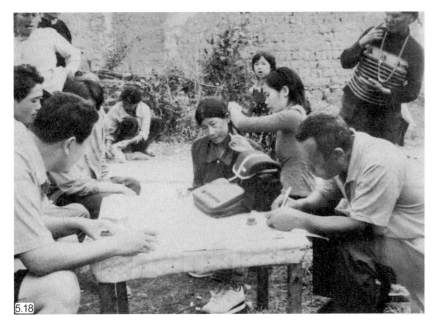

5.18

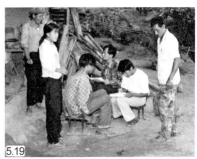

5.19

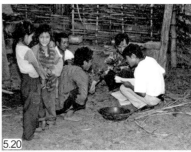

5.20

图 5.21~5.24

使用杀虫剂浸泡蚊帐和分发长效蚊帐是全球基金疟疾项目主要媒介控制措施。在全球基金项目的支持下，云南边境25县（市）重点疟区杀虫剂蚊帐覆盖率达到85%以上。

Fig. 5.21-5.24

Using insecticide treated nets (ITNs) and long-lasting insecticidal nets (LLINs) are the vector control measures of the GFATM malaria project. As a result of the support of the GFATM project, the coverage rate of ITNs/LLINs achieved more than 85% in malaria endemic areas of the 25 border counties (cities).

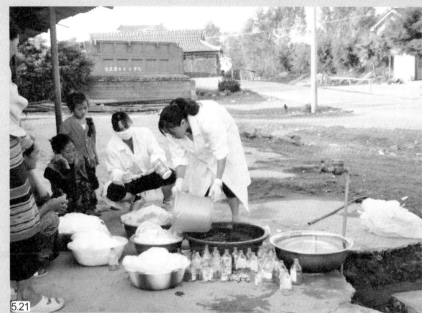

5.21

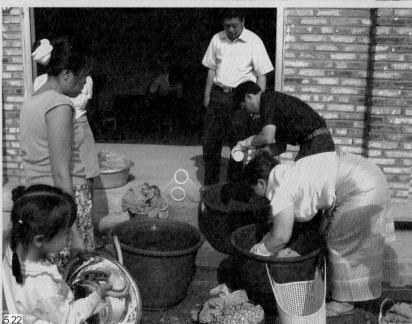

5.22

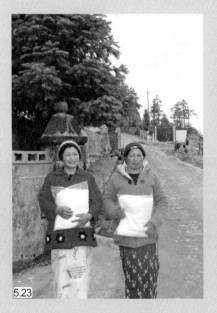

5.23

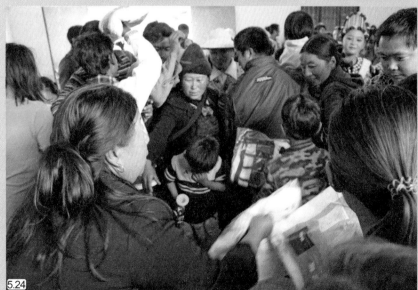

5.24

1944
1945
1946
1947
1948
1949
1950 1950
1951
1952
1953
1954
1955 1955
1956
1957
1958
1959
1960
1961
1962
1963
1964
1965
1966
1967
1968
1969
1970 1970
1971
1972
1973
1974
1975
1976
1977
1978
1979
1980
1981
1982
1983
1984
1985 1985
1986
1987
1988
1989
1990
1991
1992
1993
1994
1995
1996
1997
1998
1999
2000
2001
2002
2003
2004
2005
2006
2007
2008
2009
2010 2010
2011
2012
2013
2014
2015
2016
2017
2018
2019
2020 2020

第六部分
消除疟疾

Part 6
Eliminating Malaria

2010年10月23日，云南省消除疟疾项目启动会在昆明召开，将消除疟疾工作列入政府工作目标。同年12月，云南省卫生厅、发展改革委和财政厅等13个厅局委办联合下发了云卫发〔2010〕1256号文《关于印发〈云南省消除疟疾行动计划实施方案（2010—2020年）〉的通知》，标志着云南省消除疟疾工作正式启动。实施方案明确了云南省消除疟疾的总目标为到2015年，全省边境地区17个疟疾高传播县（市）疟疾发病率控制到万分之一以下，其他地区阻断疟疾传播，实现无本地感染疟疾病例；到2020年，全省实现消除疟疾目标。

云南省各级政府对消除疟疾工作高度重视，在省委省政府的统一领导下，成立了以省卫生厅分管领导为组长，13个部门为成员单位的云南省消除疟疾工作领导协调小组，负责消除疟疾协调工作及政策制定。领导协调小组下设办公室和云南消除疟疾技术指导组，负责全省消除疟疾工作方针、政策、规划和措施的制定，综合协调各部门工作。全省16个州（市）及129个县（市、区）也都分别成立相应的组织机构，负责全面组织执行辖区消除疟疾的各项措施。其他各部门支持、配合卫生部门的工作。

图 6.1

云南省消除疟疾项目启动后，在中国全球基金国家策略项目支持下，省、州（市）、县（市、区）各级举办消除疟疾管理、技术和财务培训班，提高消除疟疾工作管理和技术能力，以保障消除疟疾工作质量。

Fig. 6.1

Closely following the launch of the malaria elimination project in Yunnan Province, in order to improve the management and technical capacity in malaria elimination activities so that the quality of the operations could be guaranteed, training courses of management, technology and finance on malaria elimination work were held at the provincial, municipal and county levels, respectively, under the support of the GFATM with China National Strategy Application Project.

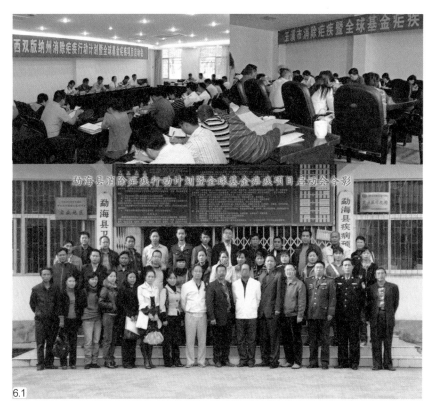

6.1

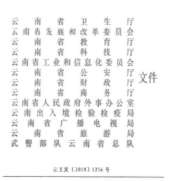
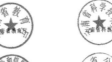
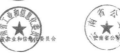
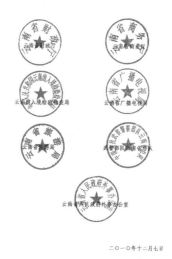

6.2

图 6.2

原省卫生厅、发展改革委和财政厅等13个厅局委办2010年12月联合下发了云卫发〔2010〕1256号文《关于印发〈云南省消除疟疾行动计划实施方案（2010—2020年）〉的通知》。

Fig. 6.2

In December 2010, thirteen departments and bureaus, including the former Health Department of Yunnan Province, the Development and Reform Commission and the Department of Finance, jointly issued the *On Issuing the Implementation Programme of Yunnan Province Malaria Elimination Action Plan (2010-2020)*.

图 6.3

云南省各州（市）所辖县（市、区）疟疾流行区分类。

Fig. 6.3

Stratification of malaria areas in Yunnan Province at the start of malaria elimination action plan.

云南省各州（市）所辖县（市、区）疟疾流行区分类

州（市）	一类县（市、区）	二类县（市、区）	三类县（市、区）
德宏	潞西、瑞丽、盈江、陇川	梁河	—
保山	—	隆阳、龙陵、腾冲、施甸、昌宁	—
怒江	福贡、贡山、泸水	兰坪	—
临沧	沧源、耿马、镇康	临翔、双江、永德	凤庆、云县
普洱	江城、孟连、西盟	景东、景谷、镇沅、墨江、宁洱、思茅、澜沧	—
版纳	勐腊	景洪、勐海	—
红河	河口、绿春	个旧、红河、建水、金平、蒙自、弥勒、屏边、石屏、元阳、泸西	开远
文山	马关	富宁、麻栗坡、广南	文山、西畴、丘北、砚山
玉溪	—	元江、新平、峨山、红塔、华宁、江川、通海、易门	澄江
昭通	盐津	大关、水富、彝良、绥江、镇雄、威信	鲁甸、巧家、永善、昭阳
昆明	—	东川、禄劝、宜良	五华、盘龙、西山、官渡、嵩明、晋宁、富民、石林、呈贡、寻甸、安宁
曲靖	—	—	麒麟、宣威、沾益、陆良、师宗、罗平、富源、会泽、马龙
大理	—	—	大理、永平、巍山、南涧、祥云、弥渡、宾川、鹤庆、漾濞、洱源、剑川、云龙
楚雄	—	楚雄、双柏、牟定	南华、禄丰、武定、元谋、永仁、姚安、大姚
丽江	—	永胜、华坪	古城、玉龙、宁蒗
迪庆	维西	香格里拉	德钦
合计	19	55	55

（其中分类根据2006—2008年疟疾疫情报告数）

6.3

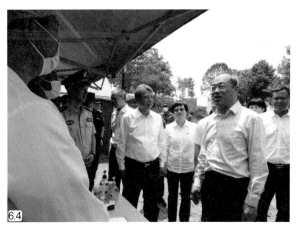

6.4

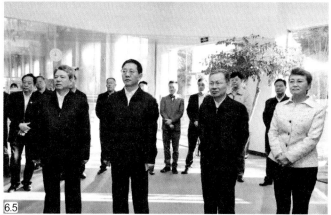

6.5

2010—2014年采取分类消除疟疾技术策略与措施。其中，一类和二类县（市、区）中的重点疟区乡镇，采取加强传染源控制与媒介防制并重的措施，以降低发病率，达到阻断传播的目的；其他二类县（市、区）以清除疟疾传染源为主；三类县（市、区）加强监测和输入病例处置，防止发生继发病例。

2015—2018年采取分类指导，加强边境防护，清点拔源的策略和措施，一类县（市、区）和二类县（市、区）中的重点边境县（市）采取边境"三道防线"策略与措施。其中，第一道防线：通过加强边境19个县（市）及其重点乡镇疟疾监测和疫点处置能力，及时发现传染源，规范处置疫点，防止发生二代病例。第二道防线：通过巩固边境68个疟疾防治咨询站，与口岸联合建立防治疟疾屏障，加强疟疾管理，开展监测，及时发现输入疟疾病例和规范治疗病人。第三道防线：通过加强对应境外边境地区合作，采取双边

图 6.4~6.10

各级领导对云南消除疟疾工作进行现场检查指导。

Fig. 6.4-6.10

The leaders from each level conducted on-site supervison and guidance on the malaria elimination work in Yunnan.

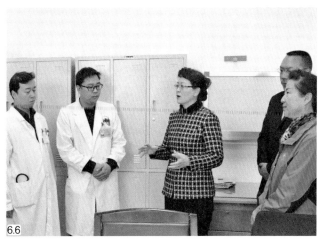

6.6

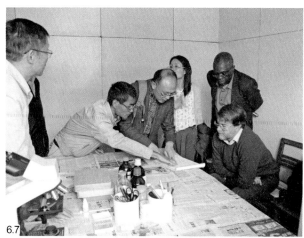

6.7

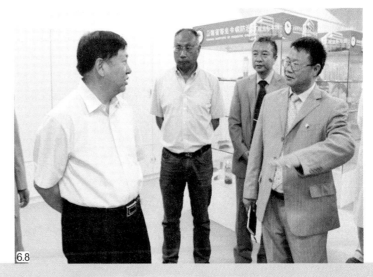

6.8

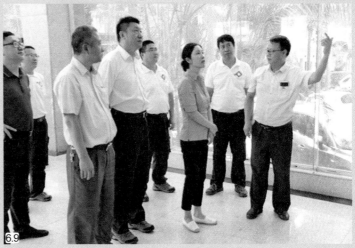

6.9

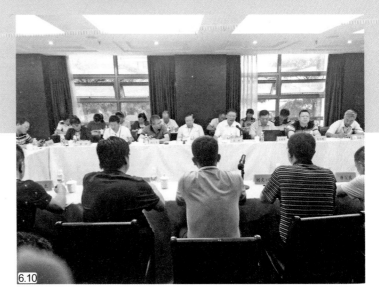

6.10

联防联控合作机制，帮助对应境外边境线一侧地区巩固疟疾防治点，提高控制疟疾能力，降低发病率，减少输入性疟疾对中国消除疟疾的威胁。

2019年起根据云南省特殊的边境疟疾防控形势，采取边境消除疟疾 "3+1" 新策略。其中，"+1" 为境外边境地区，采取的策略是联防联控合作机制，加强境外技术和物资支持，加强信息沟通，提高境外周边地区疟疾防控能力，降低发病率，减少疟疾病例输入对云南省消除疟疾的影响。"3" 中的第一道防线是指云南边境沿线2.5千米内，且对面2.5千米内有村寨或居民点的抵边村寨，采取精准研判策略，贯彻 "一村一策" 的精细化防控措施；第二道防线是指云南边境一线的抵边乡镇，建立以精细、强化的社区为基础的疟疾监测与快速响应体系；第三道防线是指在云南边境县（市）的非边境乡镇，采取以医疗机构疟疾病例监测为主，县（市）疾控中心为核心的疟疾监测和响应工作体系的策略。

通过十多年的消除疟疾工作，云南省已建立完善的疟疾监测防控四级网络，省、州（市）、县（市、区）、乡（镇）均有专人负责消除疟疾工作，并有完整的归档工作资料；医疗机构将 "三热" 病人的疟原虫筛查列入常规检查项目；输入性病例从2010年的1 136例减少到2020年的163例。自2015年5月报告最后一例本地感染恶性

图 6.12~6.13

2010年以来，云南省各地严格按照《消除疟疾技术方案》开展疟疾个案流调和疫情处置。图6.12为2015年施甸县疾控中心到旧城乡开展疟疾疫点处置。图6.13为2016年省、州（市）、县（市、区）消除疟疾驻点工作组在盈江县那邦镇开展疟疾疫点处置。

Fig. 6.12-6.13

Since 2010, all parts of Yunnan Province have carried out epidemiological investigation and response to malaria cases following *the Technical Standard Operation Procedure for Malaria Elimination*. Fig. 6.12 shows Shidian County CDC carrying out response activity to malaria cases at Jiucheng Township in 2015. Fig. 6.13 shows the joint provincial, prefecture and county team carrying out response activity to malaria cases in Nabang Town, Yingjiang County in 2016.

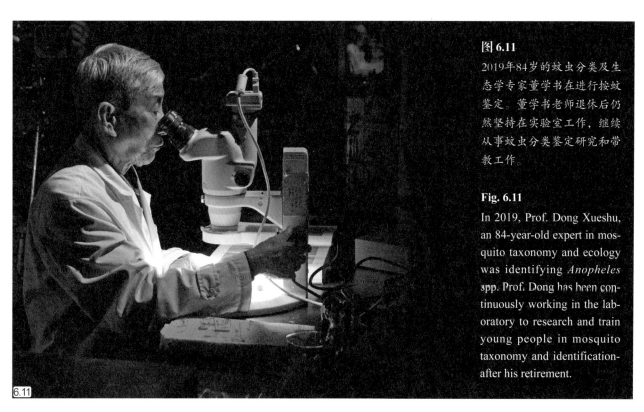

6.11

图 6.11

2019年84岁的蚊虫分类及生态学专家董学书在进行按蚊鉴定。董学书老师退休后仍然坚持在实验室工作，继续从事蚊虫分类鉴定研究和带教工作。

Fig. 6.11

In 2019, Prof. Dong Xueshu, an 84-year-old expert in mosquito taxonomy and ecology was identifying *Anopheles* spp. Prof. Dong has been continuously working in the laboratory to research and train young people in mosquito taxonomy and identification after his retirement.

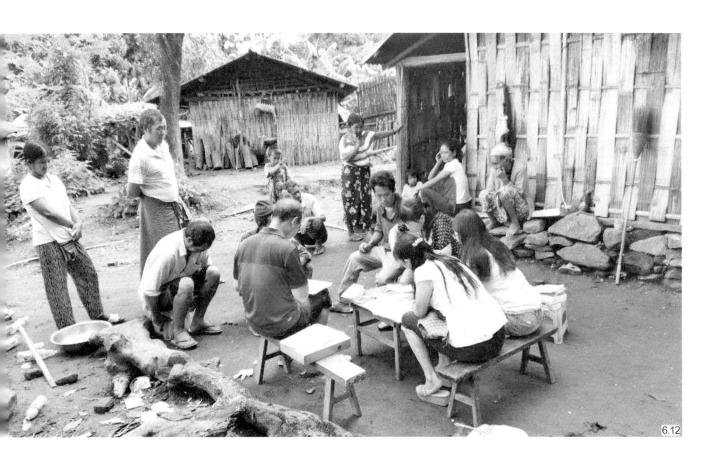

6.12

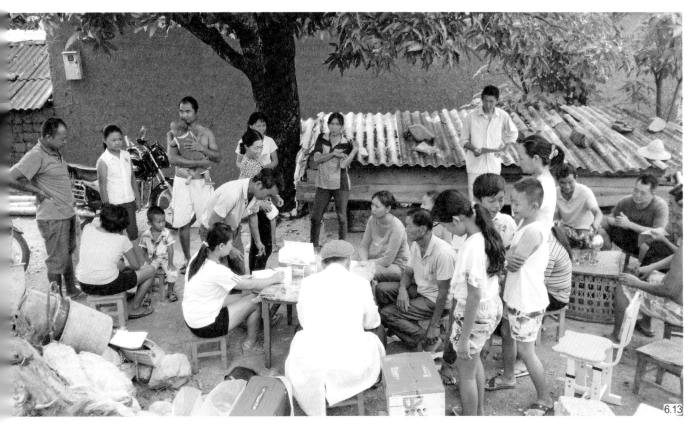

6.13

疟病例，2016年报告最后一例本地感染间日疟病例以来，至今无本地感染疟疾病例报告和继发病例发生，实现了云南省消除疟疾的目标。2020年1月，通过了国家消除疟疾技术评估；2020年6月，通过了国家消除疟疾终审评估；2021年5月17—23日，代表国家接受了世界卫生组织（WHO）消除疟疾评估专家组现场认证评价；2021年6月30日，格林尼治标准时间零点，WHO正式宣布"中国通过消除疟疾认证"。

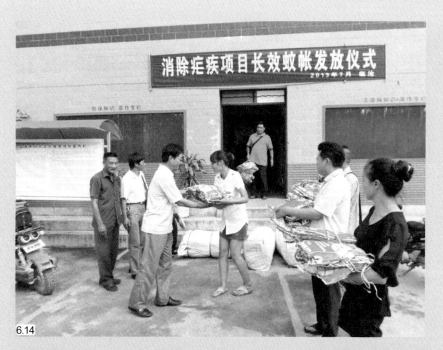

6.14

图 6.14

2013年7月，原云南省寄生虫病防治所杨恒林所长在临沧市耿马县孟定镇向当地村民发放长效蚊帐。

Fig. 6.14

In July 2013, Yang Henglin, former director of Yunnan Institute of Parasitic Diseases was distributing LLINs to local villagers in Mengding Town, Gengma County, Lincang Municipality.

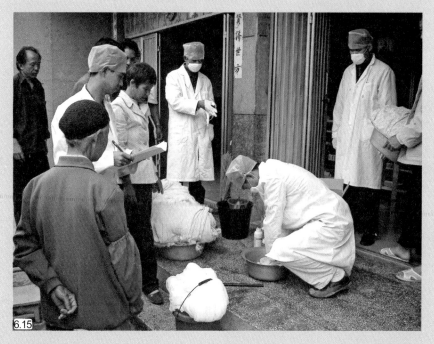

6.15

图 6.15

2011年，保山市隆阳区疾控中心疟疾防控人员指导当地村民用杀虫剂浸泡蚊帐。

Fig. 6.15

In 2011, the technical personnel of malaria control from Longyang District Center for Disease Control and Prevention, Baoshan Municipality were training local villagers to dip bed nets with insecticides.

图 6.16

2014年8月，云南省寄生虫病防治所赵晓涛和吴超医师在盈江县那邦镇指导杀虫剂的配制和滞留喷洒。

Fig. 6.16

In August 2014, Dr. Zhao Xiaotao and Wu Chao from Yunnan Institute of Parasitic Diseases were guiding indoor residual spraying with insecticides in Nabang Town, Yingjiang County.

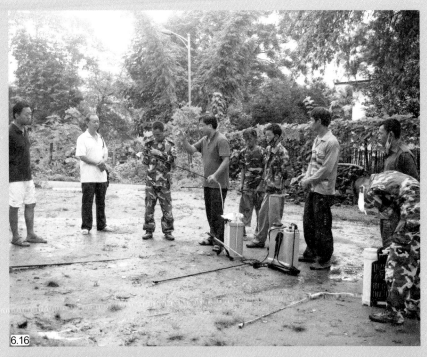
6.16

图 6.17

2017年9月，云南省寄生虫病防治所王学忠副主任医师带领年轻同志在盈江县开展传疟媒介幼虫调查。

Fig. 6.17

In September 2017, Dr. Wang Xuezhong from Yunnan Institute of Parasitic Diseases was organizing and training young colleagues to carry out investigation of malaria vector larvae in Yingjiang County.

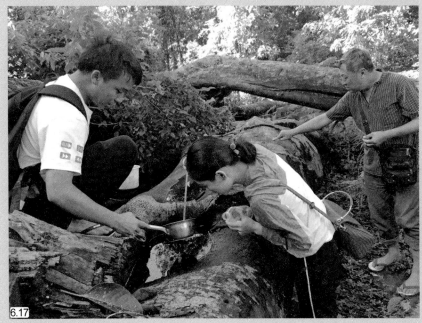
6.17

The launching meeting of malaria elimination project in Yunnan Province was held in Kunming on 23 October, 2010. Malaria elimination was put into the government's work goals. In December of the same year, 13 departments and bureaus including the former Health Department of Yunnan Province, the Development and Reform Commission and the Department of Finance jointly issued the *Notification on Issuing the Implementation Programme of Yunnan Province Malaria Elimination Action Plan (2010-2020)*, marking the official launch of malaria elimination work in Yunnan Province. The protocol set up the overall clear goals for malaria elimination in Yunnan Province: by 2015, annual parasite incidence is to be reduced to less than 1 per 10 000 person-years in 17 border counties (cities) with high malaria transmission, and in other areas is to interrupt malaria transmission, achieving no indigenous malaria cases; by 2020, the whole province is to achieve the goal of malaria elimination.

Governments at each levels in Yunnan Province paid a high attention to malaria control and elimination. Under the leadership of the Provincial Communist Party Committee and the Provincial Government, Yunnan provincial leadership and coordination group for malaria elimination was set up with the former Provincial Department of Health as the head and 13 departments as the leadership members, accepting responsibilities for coordination and policy formulation for malaria elimination. Under the leadership, there were provincial offices and technical guidance group for malaria elimination. They were responsible for the formulation of guidelines, policies, plans and measures for malaria elimination across the Province, and comprehensively coordinated the

图 6.18~6.22
云南省消除疟疾专业技能培训图片选。2011—2019年云南省各级累计培训疟疾防控人员226 024人次，临床医生和检验人员36 870人次。

Fig. 6.18-6.22
Selected pictures on malaria elimination training activities. From 2011 to 2019, a total of 226 024 person-times of public health personnel, and 36 870 person-times of clinical doctors and laboratory personnel were trained at each level across Yunnan Province.

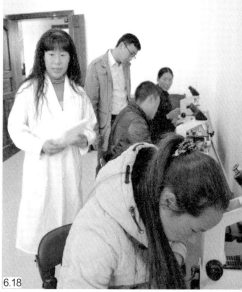
6.18

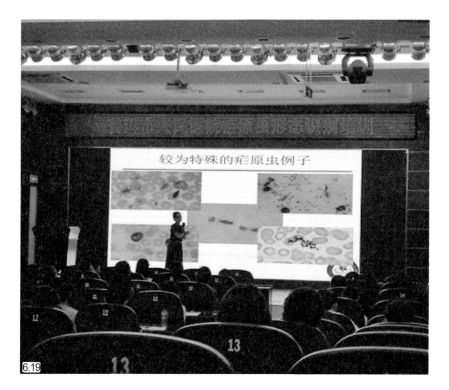
6.19

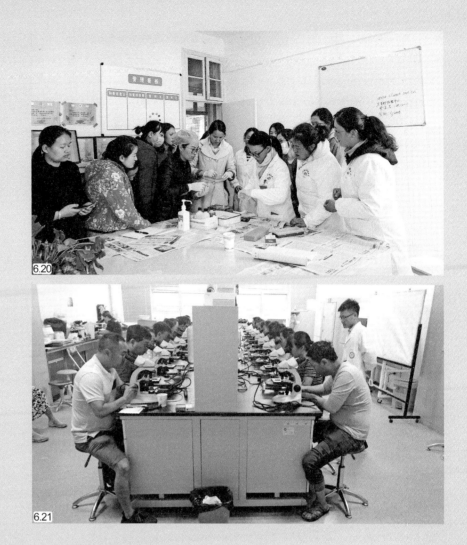

6.20

6.21

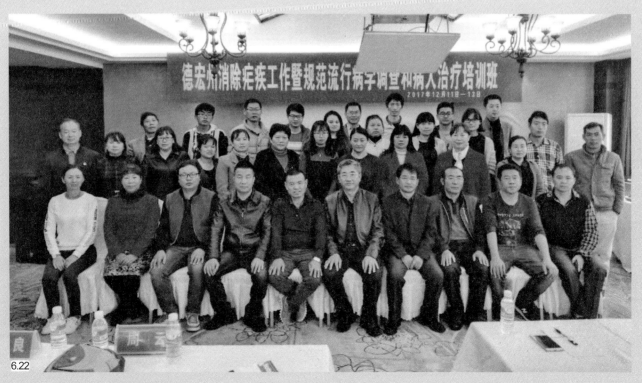

6.22

work of various departments. The same organizations had also been set up in all 16 prefectures, 129 counties (cities and districts) of the Province, which were responsible for organizing activities of malaria elimination in their own areas. Other departments supported and cooperated with the health departments to conduct interventions of malaria elimination.

During 2010-2014, different technical strategies and measures were adopted for malaria elimination in each type of malaria prevalent areas. In the main malaria endemic areas including townships of type I and II counties (cities and districts), the strategy was to strengthen the control of infectious sources and vector control, so as to reduce the incidence and interrupt the malaria transmission; in the other areas of type II counties (cities and districts), the main strategy was to eliminate the parasite reservoir; and in type III counties (cities and districts), the strategy was surveillance and treatment of imported cases to prevent malaria reintroduction.

During 2015-2018, different strategies were adopted to guide malaria elimination in different locations. The strategies of border malaria control and malaria focus clearance were strengthened. The strategy of "three border malaria lines of defense" was used in the key areas of type I and II counties (cities and districts). The first line of defense was strengthening the capacity of malaria surveillance and response in 19 border counties (cities) to detect infectious sources timely, to standardize the response of malaria foci, and to prevent introduced malaria cases. The second line of defense was consolidating 68 border malaria posts along the international boundary to screen and manage imported

图 6.23~6.26

云南省消除疟疾业务督导图片选。图 6.23~6.25：云南省寄生虫病防治所吕全、周耀武、许时燕、陈染言、孙晓东到基层进行消除疟疾工作督导。图 6.26：红河州疾控中心普舒伟科长到基层进行消除疟疾工作督导。

Fig. 6.23-6.26

Selected pictures on surveillance and evaluation activities for malaria elimination in Yunnan Province. Fig. 6.23-6.25: Lv Quan, Zhou Yaowu, Xu Shiyan, Chen Qiyan and Sun Xiaodong from Yunnan Institute of Parasitic Disease were carrying out surveillance and evaluation in the field. Fig. 6.26: Pu Shuwei, section chief of Honghe Prefecture CDC, was carrying out surveillance and evaluation in the field.

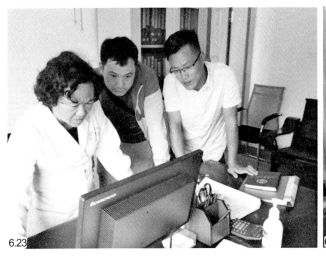
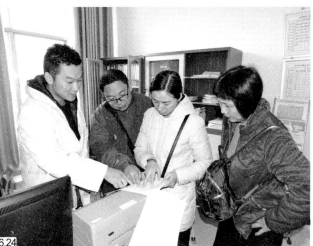

6.23

6.24

6.25

图 6.27~6.31

云南省疟疾诊断参比实验室工作图选。2016年1月—2019年12月31日，云南省级参比开展实验室复核疟原虫镜检1 196张，复核疟原虫基因检测1 196份。

Fig. 6.27-6.31

Selected activity pictures on Yunnan Provincial Reference Laboratory for Malaria Diagnosis. From January 2016 to December 31, 2019, the Laboratory re-read a total of 1 196 slides by microscopy and tested a total of 1 196 samples by polymerase chain reaction (PCR) for diagnosis quality control.

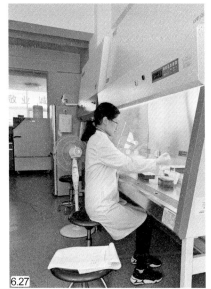

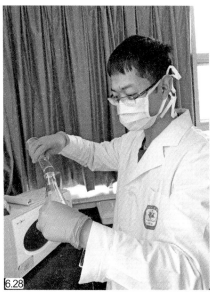

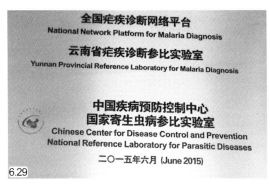

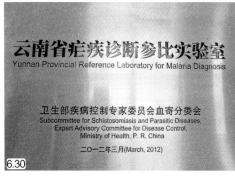

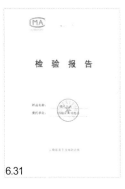

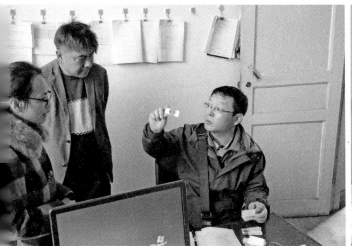

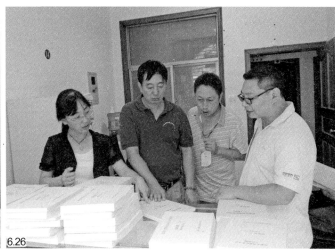

malaria cases and conducting standardized treatment of patients timely. The third line of defense was strengthening cooperation for border malaria control, by adopting bilateral collaboration mechanism to enforce malaria control measures for achieving the goal of reducing the malaria incidence and mitigating the threat of imported malaria to the malaria elimination in China.

Since 2019, targeting to the specificity of border malaria control in Yunnan Province, the "3 + 1" strategy of "one village, one policy" of border malaria control has been adopted. "+ 1" refers to the border area outside of China, and the strategy adopted is to strengthen collaboration of malaria control in the endemic areas of neighboring countries, including support in techniques, equipment and supply, information communication, training to improve the ability of malaria prevention and control. The strategy is to mitigate the threat of imported malaria cases to Yunnan Province by reducing malaria incidence in the endemic areas

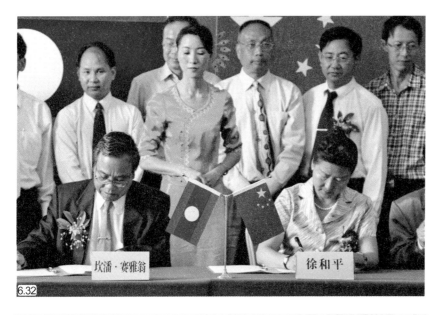

图 6.32

2013年，云南省卫生计生委徐和平副主任与老挝卫生部官员签订《中老双边疟疾和登革热联防联控备忘录》。

Fig. 6.32

Dr. Xu Heping, former deputy director of Yunnan Health and Family Planning Commission, was signing the *Bilateral Memorandum of Joint Malaria and Dengue Fever Control* with officials from the Ministry of Health, Lao PDR in 2013.

图 6.33

2019年，云南省寄生虫病防治所周红宁所长与老挝卫生部官员签订《疟疾和登革热联防联控项目合作协议》。

Fig. 6.33

Prof. Zhou Hongning, director of Yunnan Institute of Parasitic Diseases was signing the *Project Cooperation Agreement of Joint Malaria and Dengue Fever Control* with officials of Laotian Ministry of Health in 2019.

图 6.34~6.37

2018年省、州（市）、县（市、区）、乡（镇）驻点工作组赴缅甸克钦地区开展疟疾综合防控。图6.34~6.35：为当地居民开展疟原虫检测；图6.36：在当地开展传疟媒介监测；图6.37：指导当地开展媒介控制。

Fig. 6.34-6.37

In 2018, the joint provincial, prefecture, county (city and district) and township working team were carrying out integrated malaria control activities in Kachin State, Myanmar. Fig. 6.34-6.35: Malaria parasite detection for local residents; Fig. 6.36: Malaria vector investigation; Fig. 6.37: Vector control guidance in the field.

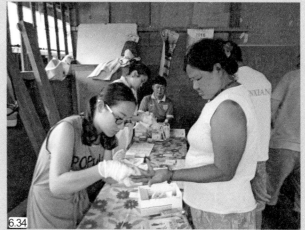

6.34

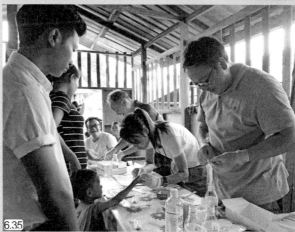

6.35

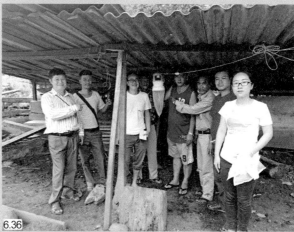

6.36

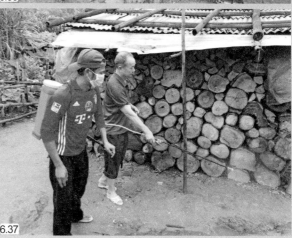

6.37

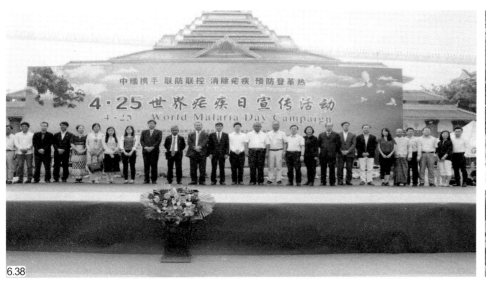

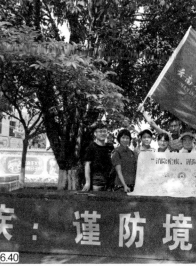

6.38

6.40

of neighboring countries. "3" is three lines of defense. The first line of defense indicates the border villages within 2.5 kilometers of our border and villages or settlements within 2.5 kilometers of the opposite side of the border. The strategy in this line of defense is to accurately judge and implement the intensive prevention and control measures by using principle of "one village and one strategy ". The second line of defense is the townships along our border, where sophisticated, enhanced community-based malaria surveillance and rapid response systems are established. The third line of defense refers to the non-border townships in border-county districts, where the strategy should strengthen medical facility-based malaria surveillance and county CDC-centered response systems.

图 6.38

2018年，中缅"4·25"世界疟疾日宣传活动在德宏州瑞丽口岸举办。

Fig. 6.38

China and Myanmar jointly held "25th April" World Malaria Day campaign at Ruili Port, Dehong Prefecture in 2018.

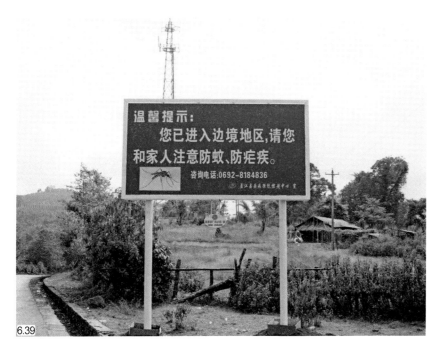

6.39

图 6.39

德宏州盈江县疾控中心在进入边境乡镇的主干道上设置疟疾宣传提示牌。

Fig. 6.39

The Yingjiang CDC set up propaganda and warning signs for malaria prevention at the border entries.

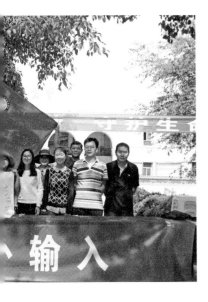

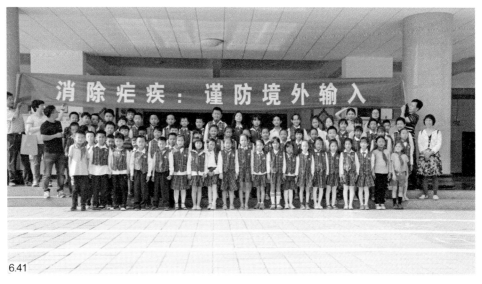

6.41

图 6.40~6.41

云南省寄生虫病防治所联合普洱市和思茅区疾病预防控制中心，2018年4月26日在思茅举办"4·26"全国疟疾日宣传活动。

Fig. 6.40-6.41

Yunnan Institute of Parasitic Diseases, the Centers for Disease Control and Prevention of Pu'er Municipality and Simao District, held the "26th April" National Malaria Day campaign at Simao in 2018.

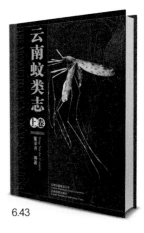

6.42   6.43

图 6.42~6.47

云南省寄生虫病防治所在消除疟疾过程中出版的书籍，包括《云南疟疾》《中国全球基金云南疟疾项目实施与效果评价》《中国按蚊分类检索》《中国云南-大湄公河次区域疟疾/登革热联防联控合作》《云南蚊类志》等。

Fig. 6.42-6.47

Books published by Yunnan Institute of Parasitic Diseases during malaria elimination, including *Yunnan Malaria*, *Implementation and Effects on Malaria Program of China Global Fund*, *Keys Taxonmia to the Anopheles of China*, *Innovative Decade of Cross-border Joint Prevention & Control Project of Malaria and Dengue Fever in Yunnan China- GMS Areas* and *the Mosquito Fauna of Yunnan China*, etc.

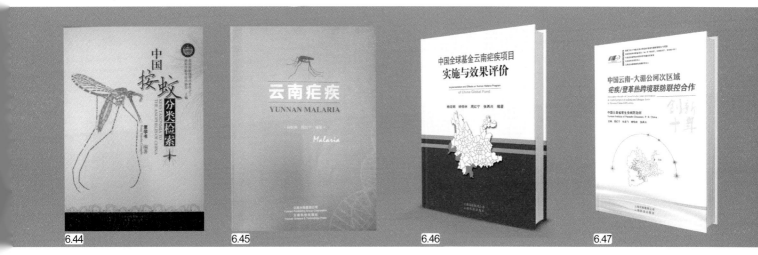

6.44   6.45   6.46   6.47

As a result of malaria elimination for nearly 10 years, Yunnan Province has established a sound four-level network for malaria surveillance and control. At each of the four levels, namely, province, prefecture, county (city, district) and township, the assigned personnel are available to take charge of malaria elimination. They have recorded and archived complete set of work data. Testing febrile patients for malaria has been included in the routine examination items by medical institutions. The number of imported cases has been reduced from 1 136 in 2010 to 163 in 2020. The last indigenous *P. falciparum* malaria case was reported in May 2015 and the last indigenous *P. vivax* malaria case was reported in 2016. Ever since, no further indigenous malaria cases have been reported, and the goal of malaria elimination has been achieved in Yunnan Province. Yunnan Province passed the national malaria elimination technical assessment in January 2020 and the final national assessment of malaria elimination in June 2020. From 17 to 23 May, 2021, Yunnan represented China to accept the on-site certification evaluation of the World Health Organization (WHO) malaria elimination certification team. WHO officially released in press that "China is certified malaria-free" at 00:01 GMT on 30 June 2021.

图 6.48~6.50

云南消除疟疾期间获奖情况。2000年以来获省部级成果奖6项，获得国家专利1项。

Fig. 6.48-6.50

Awards during malaria elimination in Yunnan. A total of six provincial or ministerial achievements and one national patent had been awarded to malaria since 2000.

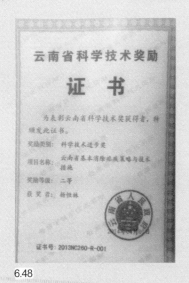

6.48

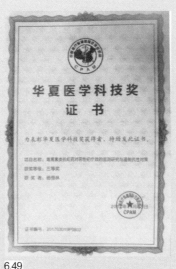

6.49

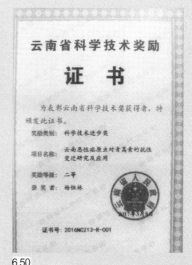

6.50

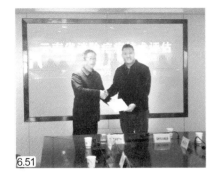

6.51

图 6.51

国家消除疟疾技术评估组组长高琪教授向云南省卫生健康委陆林巡视员递交《云南省消防疟疾技术评估报告》。

Fig. 6.51

Prof. Gao Qi, the team leader of national malaria elimination technical assessment, handing over *The Technical Assessment Report for Malaria Elimination in Yunnan* to Dr. Lu Lin, the inspector of Yunnan Health Commission.

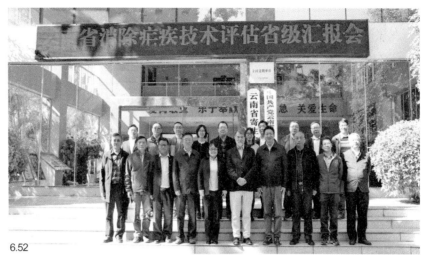

6.52

图 6.52

云南省消除疟疾技术评估省级汇报会合影。

Fig. 6.52

The group photo of provincial report meeting of Yunnan on technical assessment for malaria elimination.

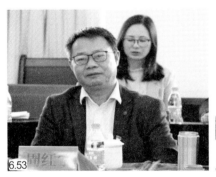

6.53

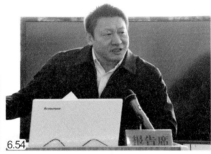

6.54

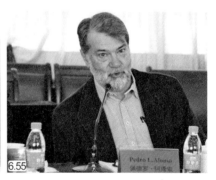

6.55

图 6.53~6.58

2020年1月15—18日，国家对云南省进行消除现场疟疾技术评估图选。

Fig. 6.53-6.58

Selected field activity pictures of national malaria elimination technical assessment in Yunnan Province from 15 to 18 January, 2020.

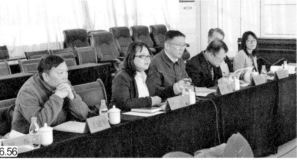

6.56

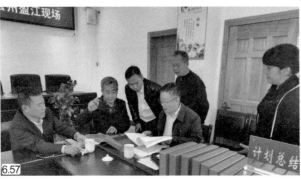

6.57

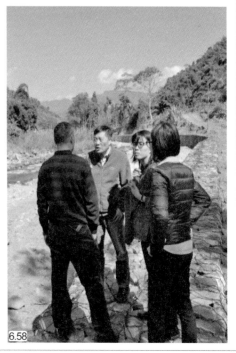

6.58

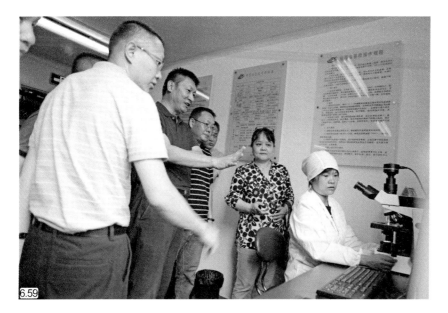

图 6.59

国家消除疟疾专家组对云南省消除疟疾进行终审评估，到盈江县疾控中心考核现场。

Fig. 6.59

During the final assessment of malaria elimination, the national malaria elimination expert team visited Yingjiang CDC, Yunnan Province.

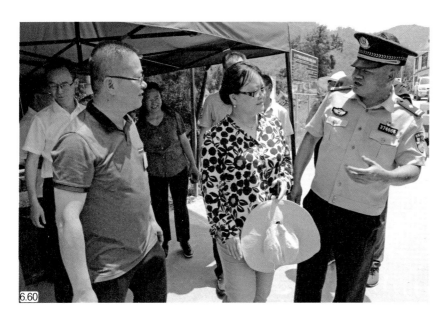

图 6.60

国家消除疟疾专家组对云南省消除疟疾进行终审评估，到盈江县那邦镇和口岸考核现场。

Fig. 6.60

During the final assessment of malaria elimination, the national malaria elimination expert team visited Nabang Town and Port, Yingjiang County, Yunnan Province.

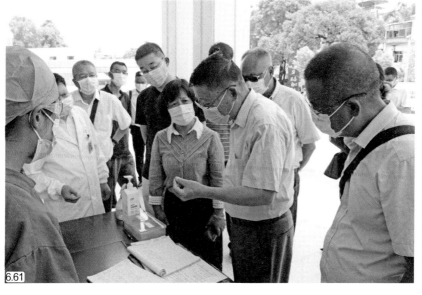

图 6.61

国家消除疟疾专家组对云南省消除疟疾进行终审评估，到耿马县孟定镇中心卫生院发热门诊考核现场。

Fig. 6.61

During the final assessment of malaria elimination, the national malaria elimination expert team visited the clinic for febrile patients at Mengding Town Central Hospital, Gengma County, Yunnan Province.

图 6.62

2020年6月5日，国家卫生健康委疾控局一级巡视员贺青华宣布云南省通过国家消除疟疾终审评估。

Fig. 6.62

On June 5, 2020, He Qinghua, the first-level inspector from Bureau for Disease Control and Prevention, National Health Commission, announced that Yunnan Province passed the final national assessment of malaria elimination.

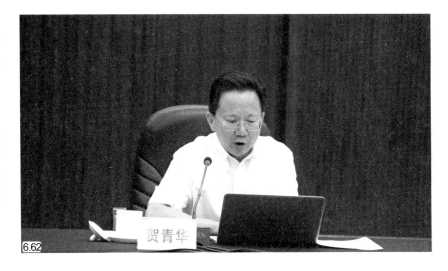

图 6.63

国家对云南省开展消除疟疾终审评估合影。

Fig. 6.63

The group photo of participants for the final national assessment of malaria elimination in Yunnan Province.

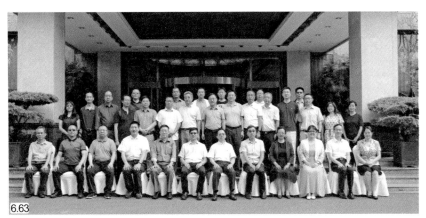

图 6.64

国家卫生健康委关于云南省通过终审评估的正式文件。

Fig. 6.64

The Official Document of National Health Commission to confirm that Yunnan Province passed the assessment of malaria elimination.

消除疟疾，是云南继消灭天花后，在公共卫生领域取得的又一重大突破，具有里程碑意义，标志着云南彻底摘掉了"瘴疫之区"的帽子，成绩来之不易，可喜可贺！谨向为全省消除疟疾目标付出艰辛努力的同志们表示感谢和慰问！

希望各地、有关部门始终坚持以人民为中心的发展思想，把维护人民健康放在更加重要的位置，以实施推进爱国卫生专项行动和"双提升"工程为契机，着力提高全省公共卫生和疾病预防控制能力，持续巩固消除疟疾成果，努力提升全省人民健康水平，为推进健康云南建设作出新贡献。

阮成发

2020年7月2日

6.65

图 6.65

原云南省省长阮成发批示指出：消除疟疾，是云南继消灭天花后，在公共卫生领域取得的又一重大突破，具有里程碑意义，标志着云南彻底摘掉了"瘴疫之区"的帽子，成绩来之不易，可喜可贺！谨向为全省消除疟疾目标付出艰辛努力的同志表示感谢和慰问！希望各地、有关部门始终坚持以人民为中心的发展思想，把维护人民健康放在更加重要的位置，以实现推进爱国卫生专项行动和"双提升"工程为契机，着力提高全省公共卫生和疾病预防控制能力，持续巩固消除疟疾成果，努力提升全省人民健康水平，为推进健康云南建设作出新贡献。

Fig. 6.65

Ruan Chengfa, former governor of Yunnan Province, pointed out in his instructions: Malaria elimination is another major breakthrough in public health after smallpox eradication. It's a milestone marking that Yunnan has completely removed the label of "Endemic Area of Malaria". The achievement is not easy, and deserves to be congratulated. We would like to express gratitude to those who have made arduous efforts to eliminate malaria in the whole province. Hoping each relevant department at each location and level will always adhere to the people-centered development principle, continuously put people's health in a more important position, take the implementation of the special action to promote Patriotic Health and the "Double Improvement" Project as an opportunity, strive to improve the province's public health and disease prevention and control ability, continue to consolidate the achievements of malaria elimination, strive to improve the capacity in public health and disease prevention and control across the Province, maintain the achievement of malaria elimination, make further efforts to improve the health of the people and make new contributions to "Healthy Yunnan".

图 6.66~6.73

WHO消除疟疾评估专家组，于2021年5月17—23日在云南进行了中国消除疟疾现场认证。云南省人民政府李玛琳副省长、云南省卫生健康委陆林副主任等相关领导莅临认证现场。WHO专家先后对云南省寄生虫病防治所，昆明海关，普洱孟连县、德宏盈江县疾控中心、县人民医院、乡镇卫生院、村卫生室等卫生机构消除疟疾工作进行现场认证，对云南消除疟疾工作和成绩给予了高度评价。

Fig. 6.66-6.73

From 17 to 23 May, 2021, the WHO malaria elimination certification team conducted on-site malaria elimination certification in Yunnan. Li Malin, vice governor of Yunnan provincial government and Lu Lin, the deputy director of Yunnan Provincial Health Commission and other relevant leaders attended the certification. The WHO expert team visited health facilities, including Yunnan Institute of parasitic diseases, Kunming Customs, Menglian County, Dehong Yingjiang County CDC, the County People's Hospital, the Township Hospital and the Village Health Posts, to conduct the field certification activities. During the certification process, the WHO team highly appreciated Yunnan's work and achievements of malaria elimination.

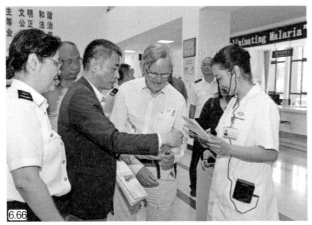

6.66

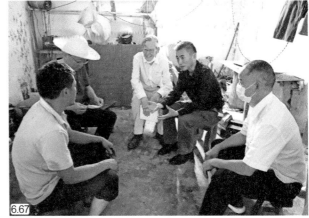

6.67

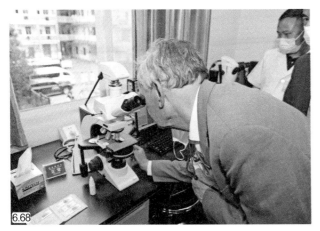

6.68

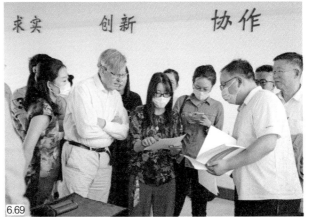

6.69

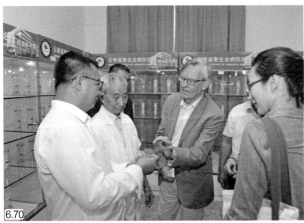

6.70

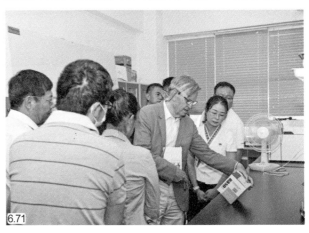

6.71

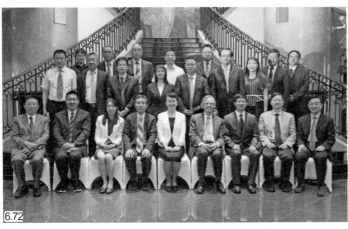

6.72

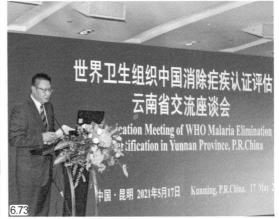

6.73

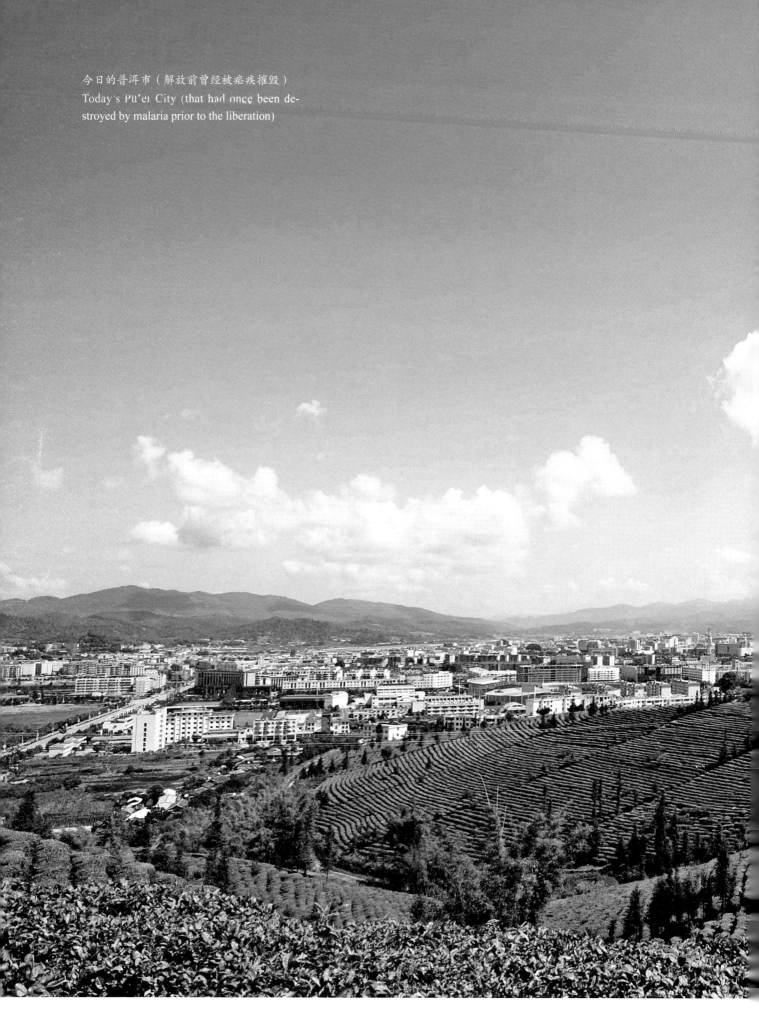

今日的普洱市（解放前曾经被疟疾摧毁）
Today's Pu'er City (that had once been destroyed by malaria prior to the liberation)

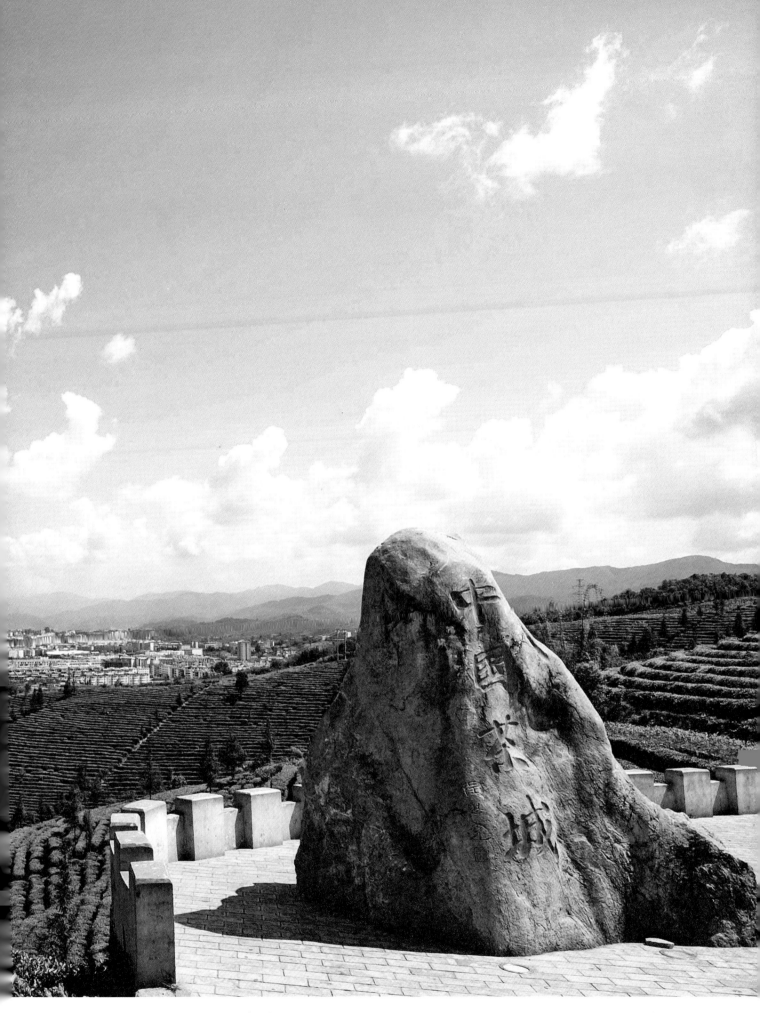

附录
Appendix

1. 1957年以来历届所级党支部/党委（纪委）任职人员清单

届次	姓名	性别	职务	任职开始时间
第一届	陈绍敏	男	党支部书记	1957年5月
第二届	付桂臣	男	党支部书记	1958年2月
	黄耀宗	男	党支部副书记	1972年12月
第三届	付桂臣	男	党支部书记	1972年12月
第四届	卫全达	男	党支部书记	1981年5月
第五届	卢树德	男	党支部书记	1983年10月
	文　华	男	党支部副书记	1983年10月
第六届	朱德福	男	党支部书记	1991年4月
	周新文	男	党支部副书记	1995年9月
第七届	周新文	男	党委书记	2002年5月
	张志勇	男	纪委书记	2011年4月
第八届	张志勇	男	党委书记	2015年8月
	杜龙飞	男	纪委书记	2016年11月

1. The Name List of Successive Party Branches/Committees (Discipline Inspection Commissions) of Yunnan Institute of Parasitic Diseases since 1957

Stage	Name	Gender	Position	Onset time
Stage 1	Chen Shaomin	Male	Branch Secretary of the CPC	May 1957
Stage 2	Fu Guichen	Male	Branch Secretary of the CPC	February 1958
Stage 2	Huang Yaozong	Male	Deputy Branch Secretary of the CPC	December 1972
Stage 3	Fu Guichen	Male	Branch Secretary of the CPC	December 1972
Stage 4	Wei Quanda	Male	Branch Secretary of the CPC	May 1981
Stage 5	Lu Shude	Male	Branch Secretary of the CPC	October 1983
Stage 5	Wen Hua	Male	Deputy Branch Secretary of the CPC	October 1983
Stage 6	Zhu Defu	Male	Branch Secretary of the CPC	April 1991
Stage 6	Zhou Xinwen	Male	Deputy Branch Secretary of the CPC	September 1995
Stage 7	Zhou Xinwen	Male	Secretary of the CPC	May 2002
Stage 7	Zhang Zhiyong	Male	Secretary of the CPC Discipline Inspection Commission	April 2011
Stage 8	Zhang Zhiyong	Male	Secretary of the CPC	August 2015
Stage 8	Du Longfei	Male	Secretary of the CPC Discipline Inspection Commission	November 2016

2. 1957年以来历届所级行政班子任职人员清单

届次	姓名	性别	职务	任职开始时间
任命	付桂臣	男	所长	1958年2月
	黄耀宗	男	副所长	1964年3月
"文革"核心小组任命	付桂臣	男	主任	1968年9月
	黄耀宗	男	副主任	1972年12月
	文 华	男	组长	1967年5月
	张彦正	男	组长	1967年9月
	朱开陈	男	副主任	1968年9月
	李春堂	男	主任	1969年2月
	陈文才	男	副主任	1969年2月
	郑兴安	男	主持工作	1970年11月
	付桂臣	男	主任	1972年12月
	黄耀宗	男	副主任	1972年12月
	王绍通	男	副主任	1973年12月
	卫全达	男	副主任	1977年8月
第一届	黄耀宗	男	副所长	1981年5月
	卫全达	男	副所长	1981年5月
第二届	黄耀宗	男	所长	1983年10月
	李学忠	男	副所长	1983年10月
第三届	李学忠	男	所长	1987年11月
	车立刚	男	副所长	1987年12月
第四届	车立刚	男	所长	1991年4月
	杨 芑	男	副所长	1991年4月
	张再兴	男	副所长	1991年9月
	张国森	男	副所长	1991年9月

届次	姓名	性别	职务	任职开始时间
第五届	杨　煌	男	所长	1995年7月
	张再兴	男	副所长	1995年9月
	杨恒林	男	副所长	1995年9月
第六届	张再兴	男	所长	1998年9月
	杨恒林	男	副所长	1995年9月
	周红宁	男	副所长	2004年5月
第七届	杨恒林	男	所长	2009年5月
	周红宁	男	副所长	2004年5月
	杨亚明	男	副所长	2010年9月
第八届	周红宁	男	所长	2015年8月
	杨亚明	男	副所长	2010年9月
	杜龙飞	男	副所长	2015年8月
	姜进勇	男	副所长	2020年12月

2. The Name List of Successive Administrative Leaders of Yunnan Institute of Parasitic Diseases since 1957

Stage	Name	Gender	Position	Onset time
Appointed	Fu Guichen	Male	Director	February 1958
	Huang Yaozong	Male	Deputy Director	March 1964
Appointed by the core of "Cultural Revolution"	Fu Guichen	Male	Director	September 1968
	Huang Yaozong	Male	Deputy Director	December 1972
	Wen Hua	Male	Team Leader	May 1967
	Zhang Yanzheng	Male	Team Leader	September 1967
	Zhu Kaichen	Male	Deputy Director	September 1968
	Li Chuntang	Male	Director	February 1969
	Chen Wencai	Male	Deputy Director	February 1969
	Zheng Xing'an	Male	Interim Leader	November 1970
	Fu Guichen	Male	Director	December 1972
	Huang Yaozong	Male	Deputy Director	December 1972
	Wang Shaotong	Male	Deputy Director	December 1973
	Wei Quanda	Male	Deputy Director	August 1977
Stage 1	Huang Yaozong	Male	Deputy Director	May 1981
	Wei Quanda	Male	Deputy Director	May 1981
Stage 2	Huang Yaozong	Male	Director	October 1983
	Li Xuezhong	Male	Deputy Director	October 1983
Stage 3	Li Xuezhong	Male	Director	November 1987
	Che Ligang	Male	Deputy Director	December 1987
Stage 4	Che Ligang	Male	Director	April 1991
	Yang Qi	Male	Deputy Director	April 1991
	Zhang Zaixing	Male	Deputy Director	September 1991
	Zhang Guosen	Male	Deputy Director	September 1991
Stage 5	Yang Huang	Male	Director	July 1995
	Zhang Zaixing	Male	Deputy Director	September 1995
	Yang Henglin	Male	Deputy Director	September 1995

Tab.2 (continued)

Stage	Name	Gender	Position	Onset time
Stage 6	Zhang Zaixing	Male	Director	September 1998
	Yang Henglin	Male	Deputy Director	September 1995
	Zhou Hongning	Male	Deputy Director	May 2004
Stage 7	Yang Henglin	Male	Director	May 2009
	Zhou Hongning	Male	Deputy Director	May 2004
	Yang Yaming	Male	Deputy Director	September 2010
Stage 8	Zhou Hongning	Male	Director	August 2015
	Yang Yaming	Male	Deputy Director	September 2010
	Du Longfei	Male	Deputy Director	August 2015
	Jiang Jinyong	Male	Deputy Director	December 2020

3.1957年以来曾在单位工作的人员名单（在编，按拼音字母排序，共238人）

毕艳	蔡璇	曹建华	车立刚	陈国光	陈国伟
陈金宝	陈梦妮	陈柒言	陈绍敏	陈文才	陈岩康
陈玉英	陈章伟	陈子龙	代世林	刀美华	邓道伟
邓秀英	邓艳	丁春丽	丁夏	董利民	董学书
董莹	杜芳芳	杜龙飞	杜尊伟	段凯霞	段伟
段志刚	付桂臣	高白荷	顾云安	关淑贞	郭丽华
郭晓芳	郭小连	果荣华	何慧	何文斌	何子圭
贺春素	洪佩辉	后晋修	胡惠仙	黄冬玲	黄凤仙
黄国珍	黄红萍	黄开国	黄荣	黄世华	黄伟玲
黄耀宗	黄煜	黄云芝	姜华	姜进勇	姜天余
金淑仙	兰学梅	雷洛田	李奔福	李昌荣	李朝文
李崇珍	李春富	李春敏	李春堂	李海珍	李华宪
李建敏	李建雄	李菊昇	李科	李丽	李连生
李露森	李曼	李梅影	李荣峰	李睿洁	李世益
李兴亮	李学忠（大）	李学忠（小）	李跃光	李志娇	李宗惠
梁荣华	廖荷英	廖开信	林志良	林祖锐	刘慧
刘行知	刘言	刘银生	刘志俞	卢娜	卢树德
卢勇荣	罗春海	罗敏杰	吕全	马继东	马家昇
马丽仙	马莲爱	马婉玲	马文兴	马肖鹛	毛祥华
娜安	倪成忠	聂仁华	彭佳	彭子秀	邱淑惠

续表

沈加员	盛次星	时桂荣	宋如生	孙淑芬	孙晓东
谭锡惠	唐烨榕	田 鹏	汪丽波	汪文仁	王恒业
王 剑	王 军	王丕玉	王绍通	王喜元	王 翔
王学忠	王雪菲	王映入	王正青	王仲陶	卫全达
魏 春	魏大勇	温明德	温明阳	温 群	文 华
吴 超	吴方伟	吴 静	吴林波	吴 三	夏 敏
夏汝良	谢 吕	熊文清	徐定一	徐 倩	徐艳春
许建卫	许时燕	许 翔	严信留	杨沧江	杨凤艳
杨海龙	杨恒林	杨 煌	杨 娟	杨克宽	杨明东
杨品芳	杨 芭	杨 锐	杨寿荣	杨兴艳	杨学礼
杨亚明	杨 宇	杨沅川	杨峥雄	杨中华	杨忠平
叶升玉	尹一杰	余 蕾	余文祥	袁灿丽	曾旭灿
张苍林	张凤仙	张国才	张国森	张红琳	张建萍
张丕伟	张琼丽	张彦正	张一元	张宜萱	张有林
张再兴	张志勇	张祖顺	章祖庆	赵春星	赵声能
赵为一	赵晓涛	赵 一	赵媛贞	郑敬津	郑太乙
郑兴安	郑宇婷	郑祖佑	周 宝	周宝祥	周翠珍
周红宁	周怀仙	周懋蓉	周 升	周新文	周兴武
周耀武	周子悠	朱德福	朱国君	朱 锦	朱开陈
朱丽华	朱 莹	朱兆鸿	字金荣		

3. The Personnel Name List of Yunnan Institute of Parasitic Diseases since 1957 (A total of 238 since the establishment, in alphabetic order)

Bi Yan	Cai Xuan	Cao Jianhua	Che Ligang	Chen Guoguang	Chen Guowei
Chen Jinbao	Chen Mengni	Chen Qiyan	Chen Shaomin	Chen Wencai	Chen Yankang
Chen Yuying	Chen Zhangwei	Chen Zilong	Dai Shilin	Dao Meihua	Deng Daowei
Deng Xiuying	Deng Yan	Ding Chunli	Ding Xia	Dong Limin	Dong Xueshu
Dong Ying	Du Fangfang	Du Longfei	Du Zunwei	Duan Kaixia	Duan Wei
Duan Zhigang	Fu Guichen	Gao Baihe	Gu Yun'an	Guan Shuzhen	Guo Lihua
Guo Xiaofang	Guo Xiaolian	Guo Ronghua	He Hui	He Wenbin	He Zigui
He Chunsu	Hong Peihui	Hou Jinxiu	Hu Huixian	Huang Dongling	Huang Fengxian
Huang Guozhen	Huang Hongping	Huang Kaiguo	Huang Rong	Huang Shihua	Huang Weiling
Huang Yaozong	Huang Yu	Huang Yunzhi	Jiang Hua	Jiang Jinyong	Jiang Tianyu
Jin Shuxian	Lan Xuemei	Lei Luotian	Li Benfu	Li Changrong	Li Chaowen
Li Chongzhen	Li Chunfu	Li Chunmin	Li Chuntang	Li Haizhen	Li Huaxian
Li Jianmin	Li Jianxiong	Li Jusheng	Li Ke	Li Li	Li Liansheng
Li Lusen	Li Man	Li Meiying	Li Rongfeng	Li Ruijie	Li Shiyi
Li Xingliang	Li Xuezhong(S)	Li Xuezhong(J)	Li Yueguang	Li Zhijiao	Li Zonghui
Liang Ronghua	Liao Heying	Liao Kaixin	Lin Zhiliang	Lin Zurui	Liu Hui
Liu Xingzhi	Liu Yan	Liu Yinsheng	Liu Zhiyu	Lu Na	Lu Shude
Lu Yongrong	Luo Chunhai	Luo Minjie	Lü Quan	Ma Jidong	Ma Jiasheng
Ma Lixian	Ma Lian'ai	Ma Wanling	Ma Wenxing	Ma Xiaokun	Mao Xianghua
Na An	Ni Chengzhong	Nie Renhua	Peng Jia	Peng Zixiu	Qiu Shuhui

Tab.3 (continued)

Shen Jiayuan	Sheng Cixing	Shi Guirong	Song Rusheng	Sun Shufen	Sun Xiaodong
Tan Xihui	Tang Yerong	Tian Peng	Wang Libo	Wang Wenren	Wang Hengye
Wang Jian	Wang Jun	Wang Piyu	Wang Shaotong	Wang Xiyuan	Wang Xiang
Wang Xuezhong	Wang Xuefei	Wang Yingru	Wang Zhengqing	Wang Zhongtao	Wei Quanda
Wei Chun	Wei Dayong	Wen Mingde	Wen Mingyang	Wen Qun	Wen Hua
Wu Chao	Wu Fangwei	Wu Jing	Wu Linbo	Wu San	Xia min
Xia Ruliang	Xie Lü	Xiong Wenqing	Xu Dingyi	Xu Qian	Xu Yanchun
Xu Jianwei	Xu Shiyan	Xu Xiang	Yan Xinliu	Yang Cangjiang	Yang Fengyan
Yang Hailong	Yang Henglin	Yang Huang	Yang Juan	Yang Kekuan	Yang Mingdong
Yang Pinfang	Yang Qi	Yang Rui	Yang Shourong	Yang Xingyan	Yang Xueli
Yang Yaming	Yang Yu	Yang Yuanchuan	Yang Zhengxiong	Yang Zhonghua	Yang Zhongping
Ye Shengyu	Yin Yijie	Yu Lei	Yu Wenxiang	Yuan Canli	Zeng Xucan
Zhang Canglin	Zhang Fengxian	Zhang Guocai	Zhang Guosen	Zhang Honglin	Zhang Jianping
Zhang Piwei	Zhang Qiongli	Zhang Yanzheng	Zhang Yiyuan	Zhang Yixuan	Zhang Youlin
Zhang Zaixing	Zhang Zhiyong	Zhang Zushun	Zhang Zuqing	Zhao Chunxing	Zhao Shengneng
Zhao Weiyi	Zhao Xiaotao	Zhao Yi	Zhao Yuanzhen	Zheng Jingjin	Zheng Taiyi
Zheng Xing'an	Zheng Yuting	Zheng Zuyou	Zhou Bao	Zhou Baoxiang	Zhou Cuizhen
Zhou Hongning	Zhou Huaixian	Zhou Maorong	Zhou Sheng	Zhou Xinwen	Zhou Xingwu
Zhou Yaowu	Zhou Ziyou	Zhu Defu	Zhu Guojun	Zhu Jin	Zhu Kaichen
Zhu Lihua	Zhu Ying	Zhu Zhaohong	Zi Jinrong		

后　记

2020年6月5日，国家宣布云南省通过消除疟疾终审评估，标志着曾经疟疾流行最严重、消除最困难的云南，经过近70年的不懈努力，与全国同步实现了消除疟疾目标。2021年5月17—23日，云南作为中国向WHO申请国家消除疟疾认证后被专家组抽取的四个省份之一，接受了WHO消除疟疾评估专家组对中国消除疟疾的评估。2021年6月30日，WHO向全球正式宣布中国无疟疾的报告。这也是云南省在公共卫生领域中取得的伟大成就，凝聚了新中国成立以来几代从事疟疾防治、研究的专业技术人员和广大基层卫生人员的心血，是他们认真贯彻预防为主卫生工作方针，全面落实各项防治措施的结果。在长期的疟疾防治工作中，他们不畏感染疟疾的危险，深入农村和疫区，牢记使命，以奋力拼搏和无私奉献的精神铸就了驱除千年瘴疠，保障人民健康的历史丰碑！

云南省虽然实现了阻断疟疾传播，无本地感染疟疾病例的目标，但云南省特殊的地理条件，决定了输入性疟疾的威胁将长期存在，防止输入性疟疾所引起的再传播的任务仍然十分艰巨。必须在巩固现有省、州（市）、县（市、区）多层次、立体化防控成效基础上，着眼未来，建立长效机制，持续保障组织机构、人员队伍、专项经费等的投入。继续贯彻执行疟疾防控和消除疟疾的策略和措施，加强重点人群保护和监测，提升医疗机构疟疾诊治能力，以及疾控机构疟疾流行病学个案调查和疫点处置能力，提高预警机制及突发疫情应急处置能力，防止出现疟疾疫情反复。同时按照国家《防止疟疾输入再传播管理办法》要求，继续做好各项监测，有效开展防止疟疾输入再传播的联防联控工作，继续开展跨境疟疾防控合作，降低境外疟疾输入风险，杜绝输入疟疾引起的继发传播，保证全省无本地感染疟疾病例，持续巩固消除疟疾成果。

国家卫生行政部门领导、疟疾防治专业机构领导和专家，历来关心和大力支持云南省疟疾防治和消除工作，并提供了经费保障和技术支持。通过在云南建立国家消除疟疾试点，开展科学研究和技术培训，提高了云南各级疟疾防治的能力和技术水平。同时，云南省疟疾防治与消除疟疾工作得到了国家消除疟疾技术专家组、兄弟省（市）领导、专家和同行们的大力支持，在此表示感谢！

在此，特别感谢世界卫生组织、全球基金会对云南控制和消除疟疾的大力支持，正是因为有大家的共同努力，云南省才实现了消除疟疾的目标。

Afterword

On June 5, 2020, the leader of National Health Commission announced that Yunnan Province had passed the national final assessment for malaria elimination. The announce marks that Yunnan Province, once the country's malaria hyperendemic area with the highest difficulty in eliminating malaria, simultaneously achieved the goal of malaria elimination with other provinces in China after nearly 70 years' unremitting efforts in public health. From 17 to 23 May, 2021, Yunnan, as one of four provinces selected by WHO's expert group for completing China's application for malaria free, accepted the assessment of WHO's field malaria elimination certification. The WHO officially released to the world in press that "China is certified malaria-free" on 30 June 2021. The achievement notes a great achievement of Yunnan Province in the field of public health, and embodies painstaking efforts of several generations of professional and technical personnel engaged in malaria control and research since the establishment of the People's Republic of China. It is also the result of their conscientious implementation of the health work policy "Disease prevention first" and comprehensively employment of various interventions. During the long-term process of malaria control and elimination, the health personnel overcame the threat of malaria infection to work in epidemic sites of rural areas, kept the mission in mind, and their hard work and selfless dedication established a historical monument of malaria elimination. Their efforts in protecting people's health through eliminating malaria will be prevalent for thousands of years.

Yunnan Province has interrupted malaria transmission to achieve the goal of elimination. However, its special geographical conditions determine that continuous threats from malaria will persist for a long time; and the task of preventing malaria reintroduction is still very arduous. It still needs a long-term mechanism to ensure the continuous investment of personnel, special funding and others. It still needs to strengthen the three-dimensional and multi-level protection network including in provinces, prefectures and counties. The strategies and main interventions of malaria control and elimination will continuously be implemented. They include malaria surveillance and prevention among key populations, improving the hospital's capacity of diagnosis and treatment for malaria, the CDC's ability of epidemiological investigation and response for imported malaria cases, and strengthening the ability in early warning and emergency response to any potential outbreaks to prevent malaria reintroduction. At the same time, following the requirements of *The National Regulations of Preventing Malaria Reintroduction*, we will continuously consolidate the achievements of malaria elimination by effectively carrying out intensive malaria surveillance and multi-sector action to control import malaria, and continuously developing cross-border cooperation in malaria prevention and control to reduce malaria burden at the border areas of neighboring countries and we shall ensure that these strategies and interventions would prevent introduced malaria and re-establishment of malaria transmission caused in the whole province, the state of zero indigenous cases will remain, and the achievements of malaria elimination will be consolidated.

The leaders from national health administration and the experts from national scientific research institutions for malaria have supported malaria control and elimination in Yunnan Province greatly, providing financial inputs and technical support. They set up a national malaria elimination pilot project in Yunnan to carry out scientific research and technical training that helped Yunnan improve technical level in malaria control and elimination. At the same time, the work of malaria control and elimination in Yunnan Province has been strongly supported by the experts from national advisory group for malaria elimination, the leaders and colleagues from other brother provinces. I would like to express my faithful acknowledges here.

At this moment, the special appreciations would like to be given to the World Health Organization and the Global Fund to Fight AIDS, Tuberculosis and Malaria for their technical assistance and financial input in malaria control and elimination in Yunnan Province. It is because we all worked together that the goal of malaria elimination was achieved in Yunnan Province.